FALL
from GRACE

A PHYSICIAN'S RETROSPECTIVE ON THE PAST FIFTY YEARS OF MEDICINE AND THE IMPACT OF SOCIAL CHANGE

J. JOSEPH MARR, MD

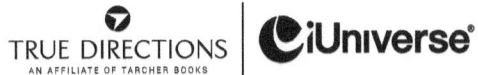

TRUE DIRECTIONS
AN AFFILIATE OF TARCHER BOOKS

iUniverse

FALL FROM GRACE
A PHYSICIAN'S RETROSPECTIVE ON THE PAST FIFTY YEARS
OF MEDICINE AND THE IMPACT OF SOCIAL CHANGE

iUniverse books may be ordered through booksellers or by contacting:

iUniverse
1663 Liberty Drive
Bloomington, IN 47403
www.iuniverse.com
1-800-Authors (1-800-288-4677)

ISBN: 978-1-4917-5485-6 (sc)
ISBN: 978-1-4917-5484-9 (hc)
ISBN: 978-1-4917-5483-2 (e)

Library of Congress Control Number: 2014921698

Printed in the United States of America.

iUniverse rev. date: 2/5/2015

To what medicine once was
And what it always has aspired to be
And the reality that is.

Where there is no vision, the people perish.
Proverbs 29:18 (KJV)

CONTENTS

ACKNOWLEDGMENTS

This book had its inception in an article published in *The Pharos* in 2014. It was an expression of my feelings about medicine in the mid-twentieth century, when I entered into it, and its current state. It also was an exploration of how medicine and we, its practitioners, came from where we were to where we are. So I must begin with a grateful bow to the more than fifty physicians who responded so favorably to the article that was the embryo of this book. They paid me the compliment of sharing their feelings and their sincere angst over current medical practice that affected them so deeply. Like me, they were perplexed over where we are now and the route we had traveled unknowingly. Even more, they and I were concerned about what society had lost. Had they not written to express their own thoughts, this book would not have been written.

The incomparable Debbie Lancaster, managing editor of *The Pharos*, generously gave of her time and talent, not only for the original article but also for this expansion. She has a delicate way of understating comments that go to the heart of the matter and cause one to rethink what he has written. She contributed greatly to the early editing process and the refinement of the manuscript. The deficiencies remain with me.

Several people were kind enough to read and comment on this book in its various iterations. Many thanks to Robert R. Kanard, MD, Anne M. Kanard, MD, James MacDougall, MD, J. Joseph Marr, III, MD, Marilyn M. Marr, MD, M. Ray Painter,

MD, Mark N. Painter, and Courtney A. Thomas, MS, RN for helpful recommendations on selected chapters. I am indebted to James House, MD for making me aware of certain references to early computing in medicine.

My wife, Marty, provided a number of creative ideas that perhaps should have occurred to me, but did not. Thanks for your help; you have done it again.

It has been a pleasure to work with the editing and production teams at iUniverse. They made a potentially tedious job a joy.

In the course of a professional life, one interacts with many people, and all have some influence. Those who influenced this book include certain important teachers, physician colleagues, research colleagues, business associates within and outside of medicine, finance and investment associates, and the patients over the years with whom I spent so many hours and who taught me so much.

INTRODUCTION

AN UNFORTUNATE THING HAS HAPPENED TO MEDICINE AND TO those of us who began to study and practice medicine in the mid-twentieth century. We were unknowingly caught up in a culture that was about to undergo significant change. The change was multifactorial, and the consequences spread themselves throughout every aspect of our society during the remainder of that century and continue to affect and afflict us today.

The change specific to medicine began quietly in the fifties as science received increasing financial support from the National Institutes of Health and similar agencies, and more medical and graduate students were educated in science. This, in due course, would bring the scientific and technological revolution of the seventies and later decades and completely alter diagnostic methods and treatment practices.

The larger and noisier change was the social upheaval of the sixties. It was a nexus of several obstructed currents of social justice that broke through as a flood and, through the late sixties and the seventies, wore away many of our anachronistic concepts and institutions. Medicine could not escape this social change and, in fact, was one of the more anachronistic parts of our society. It resisted some of the social changes while welcoming many of the technological improvements, not recognizing that the latter would inevitably carry the former with them. We welcomed, appropriately, the technology that would help our patients but were on the wrong side of history with respect to the cost and dissemination of medical care.

The turbulence caught the physician and the medical establishment off balance and kept them that way for several decades. The alterations in the reimbursement system brought about by Medicare and Medicaid and the growth of the health insurance industry created bureaucracies that regarded both patients and physicians as customers. Medevac pilots from the Vietnam War began to provide medical helicopter services; medical corpsmen from the military became physician assistants; nurses became nurse practitioners; and paramedics were trained as first responders. Over time, the character of emergency response and primary care was altered permanently. All of this was good for patient care and much of it was resisted by organized medicine.

Technological change was disruptive in most areas of our society in the second half of the twentieth century and continues to be so. The scope and pace of diagnosis were broadened and accelerated by the appearance of autoanalyzers, ultrasonography, computerized tomography, magnetic resonance imaging, and positron emission scanning, among others. The major revolution was the introduction of the microchip and digital computing. These made accumulation, sorting, and analyzing of all data progressively faster, more efficient, simpler, and cheaper. The notable exception was medical records, which is still converting to electronics even now. All of these brought with them the necessary cadre of specialists and operators, and the unanticipated result was the separation of much of the diagnostic process from the physician. Prior to these, the physician used the computer in his head to decide about diagnostic possibilities; test results accrued over days into the medical chart. New technology provided much more information in time spans measured in a few hours or less. However, the thinking process became more blunted as it became easier to get tests and then think about the diagnosis rather than the reverse. The physician was another step removed from the prolonged intimacy of the physician–patient interaction.

The adoption of good business practices in institutions that delivered medical care in the late sixties was overdue. Many of the institutions had begun as religion-affiliated charity hospitals and were in need of administrators trained in business. These new people helped control costs of medical care but could not stop the growth of costs associated with technological improvements and the care of medically indigent patients. The solution for the creeping increase in the cost of medical care from 10 percent toward 12 percent of the gross domestic product in the eighties was the entry of corporate business into medicine. Unfortunately, it behaved as large corporations do, and the creation of large for-profit health-care delivery organizations altered the dynamic of medical care enormously, disruptively, and irreversibly. Although technology and paramedical personnel had changed the dynamic of medical care, it had remained patient centered. When patients became simply items of work product, medicine lost its soul.

The nature of the change is clear from the terms themselves: medical care versus health-care delivery. The latter has a packaged off-the-shelf sense of efficiency about it. This rapid encroachment of corporate business into the management and delivery of medical care in the past two decades has altered medical care almost beyond recognition. The injection of the concept of quarterly earnings increases and shareholder dividends into patient care consigned the physician and close personal contact with patients to history. The positions of nurses changed from caregivers and patient advocates to more functionary roles. Much patient contact was relegated down to nursing personnel with a lower level of training. The activities of other paramedical personnel, whose disciplines grew up in the past thirty or forty years, changed less, as they were from the beginning focused on specific tasks. But medicine was now beginning to be practiced by a "team" and increasingly managed by middle managers, most of whom, unfortunately, had little or no immediate experience with medicine. The cost structure began to balloon from within, notwithstanding the fact that business executives had been brought in specifically to control it. The immediate response was to manage the bottom line by raising prices or premiums and cutting physician reimbursement. The consideration that a growing middle management was the issue was not addressed, nor was the fact that the executive suite and its staff had grown correspondingly. At this point, the physician had become an employee.

In January 2014, I published an article titled *Fall from Grace* in *The Pharos*, a medical literary magazine. It is published by Alpha Omega Alpha, the medical honor society, and reaches a modest but influential readership of physicians. The article dealt with the diminution of the role of the physician in society and in medicine itself over the past half century and the reasons for it. The large response from readers of the article was both surprising and emotional. Physicians usually are not given to expressing their emotions publicly. Essentially everyone agreed with the thesis yet was perplexed as to exactly how this could have happened to a group of people normally quite observant and alert. There was a strong expression of impotent rage by these responders over the demise of the personal physician who was concerned for patients' welfare and his replacement by the health-care team employed by a corporation. This anger was exceeded only by the angst of those same writers who realized that we had done much of this to ourselves. We had not paid attention to the demands and requirements of a society enmeshed in significant change and, like the privileged in the Middle Ages, had lifted the drawbridge and waited for the revolution to pass. It never did. It came and stayed, and we then were powerless to alter it.

Many responders asked why this or that facet of medical care or problem was not considered in the article; others offered opinion on how some aspects could have been addressed differently. The answer was that an article has a size limit and its purpose was to paint a picture. This book is an attempt to respond more fully to those many physicians who offered comments; to turn the picture into a mural; to examine whether medicine is better or worse (however that may be defined); and, most important, to explore whether patients are better served or not. It also is an attempt to explain to the interested public how physicians think, what motivates them, and why there is so much collective depression over medicine's current state. Physicians particularly are upset about not only what has been lost but also the fact that few in the general public understand the significance of that loss.

I agree that we have lost something very important, and this realization moved me to expand the message of that article into this book. But it is not simply the intangible of the physician–patient relationship. I believe that we have arrived at the end of an era that has lasted for centuries or, perhaps, millennia. The era was that of the shaman, the healer who, over time, became the physician. This was the person who offered advice and counsel to the afflicted, consolation when he could not cure, and cure or prevention of disease when possible. The physician was the scientist-humanist who brought the knowledge of science, the pragmatism of the doer, and an understanding of human nature to the bedside to create the art of healing. This was the historic role of the shaman and the reason that this person was respected in all societies. The presence of the physician at the bedside brought with it courage and hope to the patient. The patient had an ally, a friend, a protector, and a confidant and no longer was alone with his or her disease. This most human of interactions now has been lost. The true shame of it is that we, as physicians, have failed because we were unable to retain the best of what we brought to the bedside and meld it with the best of our new technology. That combination would have been the acme of centuries of development of medicine. Medicine could have flowered into an art that embraced the best of science while retaining the intimacy of the experience of one human helping another. Unfortunately, that was not to be. This most human of interactions was lost in the furor of change. It is that change and its effects that we will address in this book.

The prolonged contact of the taking of a history and doing a physical exam builds a relationship that is psychologically beneficial to both participants. Physicians enter into medicine because they have a genuine desire to work with people and practice both a science and an art. The technological advances removed much of the science from the direct purview of the physician, and the introduction of "physician extenders" diluted the art as well. The physician slowly evolved into an educated manager of the health-care team. The process was like vertebrate evolution itself: It is difficult to know when specific changes occurred over time. Yet, when one looks at the starting and ending specimens, the change is enormous.

Patients have benefited enormously and will continue to do so from advances in technology, new knowledge of basic science and therapeutics, and the exploitation of our expanding understanding of the genome. These will make people well who would not have been treated before, and perhaps that is more than enough to offset the loss. The goal of medicine always has been to care for people; it now is to manage sick people. The former subsumes the latter, but the reverse is not true. The latter is a more limited objective—more quantifiable, more efficient, and more businesslike.

Our society has lost something very important and does not realize it. We physicians did not stand against the philistines while there still was time to modulate the changes they brought to the health-care system. I think we really did not understand the magnitude of what was about to happen. Even if it had been explained in advance, we probably would not have believed it.

Younger physicians are not so sure about the loss. Perhaps those of us from the past fifty years are looked upon in the same way we looked upon the family doctor of an earlier era. He was beloved, honored, and respected, and he gave of his time and energy unsparingly. But he did not cure as many people as we did. Those who have come after us are just as intelligent and competent but have more knowledge and tools and will cure more people than we did. Patients, arguably, are much better off as far as diagnosis and management are concerned. How does one measure the value of an intangible?

Good medicine can persist if physicians persist in doing it. Physicians remain the patient's best advocate, and this is a function we should subsume. We are not gone; it is our model that has gone. Another has taken its place, and we should focus on improving it. No one else has the interest or ability to do so.

THE WAY WE WERE

ENTERING AN ERA AT ITS CLOSE

THE CHANGES IN MEDICINE AND ITS PRACTICE DURING THE PAST half century are well beyond anything that would have been imagined at the halfway mark of that century. The situation and the role of the physician have altered considerably. The status then enjoyed by the physician has been eclipsed by technical progress in medicine. In addition, there are many interesting and compelling scientific and technological careers available that did not exist in midcentury. They have served as magnets for younger people with high aspirations. These are the types of people who would have entered into medicine when it was the acme of careers. They have within them varying mixtures of the entrepreneur, the curious, the intellectual, the scientist, the humanist, and a touch of the pragmatist.

The science and technology that developed over these past fifty years have made it possible to have careers in information technology, astrophysics, space exploration, undersea exploration, and new sources of energy, among others. The technology of war even played a role, and an important one. Paramount in all this was the computer. It changed society and then the world, and, as it changed the world, it changed medicine. But it changed it for the better. It brought diagnostic power undreamed of and made efficient an inefficient process. It brought the recognition that medicine, unbeknownst to itself, controlled a large segment of the economy. This was a phenomenon that occurred almost by accident: As more people were born—and kept alive by sanitation and vaccination—more medicine was needed to care for them in their adult years. The costs became significant, and many people could not afford them. Physicians engrossed in the practice of a consuming art—the Magnificent Obsession of movie fame and many novels—noted but did not assimilate the societal reaction to what physicians saw only as improved methods to care for people. Soon enough, business recognized it and began to organize and manage medical care and, relatively quickly, began to profit handsomely from it.

Those of us born in the late thirties or very early forties entered medical school in the later fifties or early sixties. It was a time that I have heard described as a "Golden Age of Medicine." In surveys taken at the time, physicians were ranked second only to Supreme Court justices in public esteem. A golden age, of course, is relative to the observer. Physicians were at the top of a revered profession dedicated to the care of others, and they were almost solely responsible for the management and delivery of that care. The fact that care was very unevenly distributed and closely related to ability to pay was not a consideration. The physician wore the garb of a priest and seer; his opinions were respected, given great credence, and sought in areas outside of medicine. He was the educated person, in the broad, liberal arts sense of the term. In addition, he knew a certain amount of science, and he knew the workings of the human body and psyche as well. He was a shaman at what would be the end of the age of shamans. There is some hyperbole here, used to crystallize the image, but not too much. It was like that. Younger people thinking about careers aspired to enter medicine for reasons intellectual, altruistic, compassionate, and aspirational. The career provided a good living, but although that may have been subsumed in the career choice, it was not a driving force. The concept of helping one's fellow man had not yet become a cliché, and "My son the doctor" was a humorous descriptor but still one that many parents wished to be able to use.

Consider that medical care at midcentury truly was not too far from the time when infectious diseases ravaged populations and certain age groups—the very young and the very old. With the exception of some specific vaccinations and early antibiotic research, there had been very few real advances in medical care and therapeutics since the time of Galen. There were very real benefits to health from better sanitation, improved nutrition, and less crowded living conditions, and life expectancy was beginning to increase. But the nineteen centuries leading to our own twentieth all were about the same in terms of medical therapeutic results. There had been incremental gains in the understanding of some physiological processes and certainly a growing appreciation of the importance of public health, but the upstroke in therapeutics and disease prevention really would not take place until just before the mid-twentieth century. That was not very long ago.

Consider that we have had societies of some sophistication for about the past five thousand years; we are talking about just 1 percent of that time span. Perhaps it should not be a surprise that medical care has undergone such a metamorphosis in the past half century. What we call modern medicine moved into its adolescence at midcentury, and we know how quickly adolescents change.

There were three advances in medicine that were present at the beginning of the twentieth century and marked an inflection point that separated the century from the fifty centuries that had gone before. These were: vaccination, the beginnings of what was termed the "germ theory," and the importance of sanitation and public health in the control of disease. A second inflection point came about midcentury with the expansion of biochemistry and immunology that brought modern science into medicine. The emergence of molecular biology and the rapid expansion of technology and computers midway in the second half of the century were a third inflection point, and it is that upstroke that we are riding yet today. Note that the last two of these changes in the sophistication of medicine and medical care occurred in or around the mid-twentieth century and largely over a span of about forty years.

These changes in medicine and medical science did not develop in isolation; they were a parallel to advances in other areas. The nineteenth century had brought electricity and power grids, steel, the telephone, the telegraph, the automobile, and, as early as midcentury, the first oil well. The Industrial Revolution, building upon all of these, brought the enormous expansion of the railroads and steamships. The advent of the railroad was the first real change in locomotion since the time of the Romans. Think about that! The momentum of new ideas and the savoir faire to bring them into commercial reality provided the momentum for an enthusiastic start to the twentieth century. Much of this was on view at the Chicago World's Fair (Columbian Exposition) in 1893 and both summarized the astounding scientific and technical advances of the nineteenth century and presaged what might be anticipated from the twentieth. Despite the heroic efforts of its organizers and planners, it did not come even close to what the twentieth century would bring us.

We entered that century with an automobile that was functional but primitive, the zeppelin, and the beginnings of radio. Within ten years, the Wright brothers had made their flight; the helicopter made its first flight; Einstein published the *Theory of Relativity*; synthetic plastic, the gyrocompass, and the first sonar appeared; and William Kellogg invented Corn Flakes. At the end of the century, transcontinental flight was routine; we had walked on the moon; space travel had become commonplace; the Internet and the World Wide Web were in use internationally; the home computer had become a standard household implement; the digital cell phone had been invented; digital images had replaced film; and, as a capstone, we had invented Viagra.

VACCINATIONS AND GERMS

It was as recent as 1885 that Louis Pasteur, a polymath chemist, demonstrated to a skeptical world that rabies could be prevented by a vaccine. He was not the first to demonstrate the benefits of immunization. Smallpox immunization (variolation) was introduced into Great Britain in 1721 by Lady Wortley Montagu, the wife of the British ambassador to Turkey. That technique, which used dried material from smallpox scabs, had been practiced in the Middle East and China from the 1100s. Lady Wortley Montagu saw its value and, against great opposition, introduced it to Great Britain. Edward Jenner, a physician in Great Britain in the late 1700s, saw the clinical similarities between cowpox and smallpox and noted that milkmaids acquired cowpox in the course of their work but did not get smallpox. Accordingly, he applied the principle of variolation (from *varius*, meaning spotted) using cowpox virus—obtained from a cow named Blossom, hence the name "vaccination" (from the Latin, *vaccinus*, of cows)—to cross-immunize against smallpox. In 1796, he demonstrated that immunization with cowpox protected against a challenge with smallpox. As a result, Jenner's cowpox material replaced attenuated smallpox virus for purposes of immunization. He probably was not the first to note this inverse association of cowpox and smallpox but undoubtedly was the person who brought it into the mainstream practice of medicine.

Pasteur was well aware of all this; he already had done experiments to demonstrate the value of immunization for chicken cholera and anthrax. However, the dramatic success, using an experimental vaccine on a nine-year-old boy who had been bitten by a rabid dog, Joseph Meister, made him a hero. It also made vaccination a major tool in the medical armamentarium and catalyzed vaccine research not only in his eponymous Pasteur Institute but also in pharmaceutical companies that developed in the years that followed. This demonstration took place only sixty-five years before the midcentury we are concerned with here.

Childhood immunizations were few at midcentury, and most

of us simply acquired the diseases themselves. However, the technology and science of immunization were developing rapidly and would produce successful vaccines for polio in the middle fifties and a succession of vaccines for childhood diseases in the ensuing half century. This scientific base of biological and biochemical knowledge as applied to medicine was emblematic of other fields of scientific endeavor that would fuse the world of science to the world of medicine. The best known of these, at that time and for several decades thereafter, was the field of antibiotics.

It was Pasteur, that amazing investigator, who indirectly brought about the field of antibiotic research. He did not do any of it himself, but he created the scientific milieu that brought it about. Around 1856, he had been invited to investigate the problem of spoiled fermentation of beer and suggested, on the basis of good evidence, that microbes caused this problem. He was ridiculed by various experts, since evidence then, as now, carried little weight compared to personal conviction. In 1865, having studied beer, wine, and milk, he investigated a disease that killed silkworms and showed that it was due to a microorganism. Thereafter, he showed that chicken cholera was an infectious disease and that it could be prevented with a vaccine. Later, he did the same with anthrax.

The knowledge that diseases could be caused by microorganisms led to exploration of this issue, and medical personnel, pragmatic as they are, thought immediately of how these organisms could be eliminated. It was Alexander Fleming's observation in 1928 that a mold could kill certain bacteria that led ultimately to the discovery of penicillin. This discovery was not capitalized upon until about ten years later by Howard Florey and his research group and was first used in humans in 1941. Further work, catalyzed by the demand due to World War II, made the drug available in limited quantities by 1943. That year was only nine years before the mid-twentieth century.

The only other antimicrobial available during this time was

sulfanilamide, the progenitor of many sulfa drugs, which was discovered in 1932 and was in general use in the late 1930s. This first commercially successful antimicrobial was created by Bayer in Germany and sprinkled as "sulfa powder" on an untold number of wounds during World War II. It also was a drug that would cross the "blood-brain barrier," an anatomic and physiologic barrier that prevents many compounds from crossing from the bloodstream into the brain, and could treat some forms of bacterial meningitis, a disease that was otherwise untreatable and usually fatal. This was only about twelve years before the mid-twentieth century.

The appearance of antibiotics made it clear that chemistry could create compounds or improve on those found by screening methods. This, in turn, ushered in what would be the enormous academic and commercial emphasis on what was cheekily termed "rational chemotherapy." This was research focused on finding some biochemical reaction or series of reactions that were important to a microorganism and inhibit the process by means of a chemical that mimicked one of the components in the biochemical sequence. Infectious diseases were a main focus for several decades for two major reasons: they were endemic or epidemic in the human population and caused significant morbidity and mortality, and they were caused by microorganisms that had some metabolic sequences that differed from humans. Thus, inhibition of these reactions theoretically could be done without harm to the human host. This is somewhat simplistic, because many metabolic pathways are similar—we all are products of the same evolutionary process—and toxic reactions can occur. Moreover, the human body sometimes perceives these chemicals as "foreign" and reacts immunologically against them. When this happens, one becomes allergic to a compound and it becomes functionally useless even though it remains biochemically potent. Nevertheless, the antibiotics were perceived as "magic bullets" and served as the Holy Grail of most therapeutic agents that were to be developed later for other fields—that is, a specific action without significant side effects. This dream would prove to be elusive, if not unattainable, since it is one thing to inhibit biochemistry in a microorganism, evolutionarily distant, and quite another to inhibit a reaction in a human and hope that there was not another reaction similar to it in the same person—a fundamentally illogical hope. At that time—and to a large degree it remains true now—infections were the only diseases that could be cured by medical means. Even now, most diseases are palliated, not cured. Surgical cures are something else.

At midcentury the entry of science into medicine was in its very early stages. Our understanding of the physiology and biochemistry of humans was rudimentary. We saw the promise yet had no idea of the enormous academic and industrial operations and organizations that would arise to move medicine rapidly, and almost precipitously, into the diagnostic and therapeutic golden age of the late twentieth century. The best known example was the pharmaceutical industry or, in some respects, the academic–industrial complex. This industry was unique in its ability to focus basic science on therapeutic problems and then develop the resulting compounds for medical use. It was frowned upon by many academic scientists and physicians as being outside the academy and done for profit, but history shows clearly that it was these companies that produced many effective antimicrobials and carried both science and medicine forward in the process. The adverse effects of the profit motive would not be felt until sometime later. It was the welcomed entrance of commerce into medicine.

PUBLIC HEALTH AND SANITATION

The US Public Health Service was given its impetus in 1798 when President John Adams signed into law the Act for the Relief of Sick and Disabled Seamen. The next year, Congress expanded this to include all officers and sailors in the US Navy. The Marine Service, as it was called then, spent the next century engaged in public health, as it applied to oceans, lakes, and waterways, under the direction of a supervising surgeon headquartered in Washington, DC. This position became the surgeon general, and in 1912 the Public Health and Marine Hospital Service was renamed the Public Health Service (PHS) and its powers broadened into investigations into human diseases of many types (essentially all infectious), sanitation, water supplies, and sewage disposal. From 1930 to 1944, during the Roosevelt administration, the PHS expanded to include engineers, dentists, scientists, nurses, and physicians. Thus, as the country entered the 1950s, it had in place a government medical organization that concerned itself with the many aspects of public health. It was not an organization that was known by most citizens, nor did practicing physicians pay much attention. However, its very existence made the statement that the government had a responsibility to care for its people, and the responsibility was manifest in the PHS. This organization played an enormous role in the prevention of disease through sanitation, maintenance of clean water supplies, quarantine (when necessary), and immunization. It is difficult to overstate the importance of the PHS in the progressive development and maintenance of the public health in this country. So, at midcentury, we had a large governmental organization that practiced medicine, both therapeutic and preventive, alongside the private practice community.

THE BEGINNING OF ACADEMIC MEDICAL EDUCATION

In 1910, Abraham Flexner published a report titled "Medical Education in the United States and Canada." It was commissioned by the Carnegie and Rockefeller Foundations, with the collaboration of the nascent American Medical Association, and it quickly became known as *The Flexner Report*.

Flexner was a schoolteacher in Kentucky who had a progressive view of education that gave more importance to reasoning and experimentation and less to rote memorization. His undergraduate training was at the Johns Hopkins University, and after some years of teaching he pursued graduate studies at Harvard and the University of Berlin. He wrote a book, *The American College*, which laid out his philosophy of education and brought him to the attention of educators and, more important to medicine, to the attention of the Carnegie Foundation, which was interested in improving the quality of medical education. Although Flexner had no experience with medicine, he was well-known as an educator and was selected for this reason to evaluate medical teaching from the point of view of an educator. His task was to survey the quality of medical education in the United States and Canada and make recommendations for its improvement. He immersed himself in the literature and practice of medicine and traveled widely to gain firsthand knowledge of educational practices. His studies in Germany weighed significantly on his perspective, and he concluded that the rigorous German style of education should be implemented in America. Scientific laboratory training was to be the foundation for subsequent clinical studies; the physician-scientist was to be the model in this country. With the publication of this report, science became enshrined as the basis for medical education. It was the demise of physician-apprentice training, also the demise for many of the various homeopathic and naturopathic schools, and the end of all forms of for-profit medical training. The dramatic change in the quality of American—and indeed worldwide—medicine can be attributed to Abraham Flexner's report and its implementation at the Johns Hopkins University School of Medicine.

From his studies, Flexner selected the medical school at Johns Hopkins University as a standard. It was ahead of other medical schools of the time in that its students had received a university education prior to admission and had to pass their first two years in laboratory sciences before entering into clinical training. This was essentially the German model of scientific medical teaching. Moreover, the concept of a full-time, university-supported medical faculty became a crucial part of the model in order to eliminate the lure of combining a university appointment with a lucrative private practice. The promulgation of the Hopkins model over the ensuing years, with Flexner's vigorous support, caused it to become the standard of medical education. It remains so today.

Four facets of medical care—private practice, public health, pharmaceutical research and development, and the academic teaching of medicine—were in place and under vigorous development at midcentury. The last three were to emerge as important forces in the increasingly scientific and technological emphasis in medicine. Yet, only the first of these, private practice, was truly visible to the general public and valued for its immediate contributions to the well-being of society. The doctor enjoyed great status in the community and was revered for his medical skills, general knowledge, and learning. Medical schools and clinical faculty enjoyed significant status as well, since they were the producers of physicians, but they were less visible in the community setting.

So the entire apparatus began to grow and mature as the century progressed, and the person most visible to the public gradually became the person furthest away from the engines of change and, paradoxically, the person least likely to affect the directions medicine was taking. The practicing physician usually was reacting to new information and incorporating it into treatment plans for his patients but not guiding the direction of medicine. He was not on the scientific and technological side and not in hospital management either. As a result, or perhaps as an unintended consequence, it was the practicing physician whose position underwent the most obvious and most dramatic alteration as we progressed from midcentury toward the close.

What we term modern medicine was an infant in the 1950s and still very much in the descriptive phase when it came to research. The wider application of biochemistry and other scientific disciplines to medicine was in its formative phase and would advance rapidly as the more basic scientific disciplines themselves entered into several decades of progress never before experienced. Diagnostic technology was largely primitive, and clinical laboratories for diagnosis were in an embryonic state as well. Clinical medicine—observation, examination, and history taking—was the mainstay of diagnosis. Therapeutics had a limited armamentarium. The physician–patient relationship was strong because the physician had to spend much time with the patient, gathering information and observing progress. It was in many respects a satisfying interaction for both. Technology would change all that.

EXPANSION OF THE MEDICAL CARE SYSTEM

SOCIAL CHANGE AND ITS EFFECTS ON THE FINANCING AND DELIVERY OF CARE

A "COTTAGE INDUSTRY," AS IT RIGHTLY HAS BEEN CALLED, HAD NO impetus to look at the larger social picture. However, the advent of biotechnology, biomedical engineering, and big business affected the physician practitioner in the way the Industrial Revolution affected the many cottage industries that it eliminated. Very few people saw it coming until it was much too late. In the 1800s, the Luddites wanted to hold back the progress of the Industrial Revolution and restore the cottage industries. In contrast to the nineteenth-century reaction, in the twentieth century no one really wanted to reverse the scientific and technological progress that was introduced into medicine. It was welcomed. However, some decades later when the institutions in which medicine was practiced and the manner in which it was practiced both began to crumble and the physician–patient bond began to disappear, it was another story. When this physician–patient relationship was directly affected, there were many who wished to turn the clock back a bit, albeit in a very selective way. The loss of the patient–physician relationship was not foreseen and now could not be recovered.

There was considerable hubris among physicians at this time. We had social status, financial rewards, and the gratification of playing an important role in our society. Physicians devoted their time to patient care and paid scant attention to the institutions in which the care was delivered unless there were obvious issues of neglect or mismanagement. They also paid little attention to medicine beyond the office or hospital visits. The problems of public health and health-care delivery to the medically indigent were left to governments, municipal hospitals, charitable clinics, and the free care provided by many medical practitioners. The fact that these municipal hospitals served sometimes as superb training facilities abetted the situation. Medical schools made use of the patient populations for teaching and put faculty members in those public institutions as teaching staff. Not uncommonly, these faculty and student positions were sought after because of the excellent training offered and the freedom given to younger faculty for self-development. The university hospitals were much more top-heavy with senior faculty, and the programs were not as flexible. As a result, the care provided by university-affiliated public hospitals by those departments where there were faculty and students was quite good.

Little formal effort was made to change fundamentally the system that gave care to the medically indigent. Management and planning of indigent care largely were left to those who tried to respond to medical-social issues from a background of social work, law, or politics. These are general statements, for there were physicians and physician groups that recognized these problems of delivery of care, but the emphasis remained on indigent care provided by the public sector and fee for service with some charity care done pro bono by the private sector.

During this period, the social security program was the major social insurance system in the United States. It was designed and created under President Roosevelt as a means of providing some financial protection for people entering retirement but not as the source of retirement funds. It was considered supplemental income to assure a reasonable standard of living in the later years. However, it did not provide adequate protection for the aged against the cost of health care, because few people—about half of those sixty-five years of age and older—had hospital insurance at midcentury. Moreover, even fewer had insurance that would cover physician costs. The issue of health costs in old age—then, as now—was the same. This is the time when many of us need health care and are on fixed or inadequate incomes. A serious illness can deplete savings rapidly and bankrupt an individual or a family. The cost of health insurance when purchased in anticipation of increasing expenditures in older age was quite high and beyond the financial scope of a large percentage of the senior population. There were federal and state insurance programs, but these were restrictive with respect to both eligibility and the breadth of care that was covered. The result was that those who had no financial concerns bought medical care, and the indigent who were the most in need were helped by governmental funds. The large majority in between received care that was essentially rationed according to ability to pay.

There were other problems with the existing private insurance system. One, the costs of care could bankrupt not just the poor but also those with accumulated savings. This issue was important then, remained with us through the second half of the twentieth century, and continued into the twenty-first. It figured prominently in the debates on the Affordable Care Act (ACA) of 2009-2010. In addition, private insurance companies could and would refuse to sell insurance because of a preexisting medical condition or would terminate insurance for persons in a high-risk category. This reprehensible and unethical practice, done in the interest of maintaining a suitable profit margin, persisted through the second half of the last century and was addressed directly in the ACA. Thus, in this sector of health-care delivery and payment, little changed in more than fifty years, as capitalism controlled access to medical care. The logical consequence of all this is that many could only afford health-care insurance if they were healthy and had the funds to pay for it. This is, of course, an ideal situation for risk-averse companies that are in business to manage risk.

Although we had a medical care system that was growing rapidly and beginning to make significant gains in technology and the development of therapeutics—and an educated and financially secure oligarchy managing that system—there were very large gaps in the delivery of care. From the political and social perspective, there were too many citizens who were excluded from the system, and they demanded that it be addressed. This began with the Forand Bill in 1957; it was the first bill to propose the social security approach to health care for the elderly. It would be eight years of fierce debate until the Medicare program was enacted in 1965. The lobbying on both sides—all sides, actually, since there were many players in the game—was intense and sustained. Decisions were made that involved conflicting objectives. The basic problem was to improve quality of care and the distribution of that care without disrupting the caregiving process itself. In considering that problem, it was necessary to balance several issues: manage the expenditure of funds without managing physicians' fees; cover institutional care for a sufficient period but not create incentives for prolonged custodial care; have patients share in the costs without making those costs too burdensome; cover expensive treatment without creating an incentive to use the most expensive treatment methods; and eliminate barriers to health care without paying for unnecessary care. All of this could work in harmony only if humans were not involved.

When President Johnson signed H.R. 6675 into law on July 30, 1965, he changed the complexion of medicine and medical care in this country forever. The program had two related health insurance plans: a hospital (institutional) insurance plan and a supplementary medical insurance plan for physicians and other services not covered by the former. These were known, poetically enough, as Medicare Part A and Part B.

The "threat" of Medicare and Medicaid in the sixties caused

much of organized medicine to react strongly against what was taken as governmental intrusion into medical practice. In particular, the American Medical Association (AMA), presumed to be the spokesperson for physicians generally, lobbied against any changes in the fee-for-service practitioner model of medical care. The specter of socialized medicine was raised whenever any governmental changes were proposed. The AMA carried out a vigorous campaign during the 1950s and 1960s against the proposed Medicare legislation. This intensive opposition brought about the inclusion of the language "usual, customary, and reasonable" charges into the legislation to placate the AMA. This was reactionary and focused solely on physician reimbursement. There still was no provision of a solution to the problem of the uninsured and underserved who were ineligible for Medicare. When Lyndon Johnson brought Medicare to fruition, two things happened among physicians: First, outrage. There was much talk of "socialized medicine" and the downfall of the private medical practice model. Nevertheless, practice went on as usual, though with the realization that a major event had occurred, the consequences of which were yet to develop. Second, there was the slow realization that the medical care physicians had been providing gratis now would be reimbursed by the government. Because of these payments to physicians through Medicare and Medicaid, opposition softened. We gradually came to tolerate, and then love, the beast. The words from Alexander Pope's *Essay on Man*, intended for other situations, were never truer:

> Vice is a monster of so frightful mien
> As, to be hated, needs but to be seen
> Yet seen to oft, familiar with her face
> We first endure, then pity, then embrace.

Organized medicine positioned itself firmly against any change in the fee-for-service physician-served model and opposed subsequent, and much more recent, changes, such as the nationwide trend for medical clinics in supermarkets, drugstores, or other establishments. The opposition was based upon a presumed conflict of interest on the part of the provider organization and concern about the quality of care. Both of these concerns were justifiable but largely unproven. Many of these innovations clearly were and are methods of increasing revenue, but they also are a means of bringing medical care to places more immediate and convenient to the people who need it and at a lower cost. These positions taken by organized medicine put it squarely against the tides of change when the time came.

All of this did nothing to burnish organized medicine's image as the spokesperson for medicine. It was more concerned with what it saw as potential or real economic loss to medical practitioners rather than better medical care for the people of the country. These very visible positions offered no good alternatives in times that demanded change. Concurrently, people who felt disenfranchised from good medical care—much of the general population—slowly were deciding that medical care might just be a right rather than a privilege, particularly in the wealthiest nation on earth.

Whatever the feelings of many physicians might have been, the image of the physician in the mind of the public was compromised. The physician as healer and comforter began to fade as the physician as seeker of economic gain took its place. Again, this is general statement but it was a concept widely held in our population. This, of course, provided a very useful target for politicians as the cost of health care continued to rise.

Let us consider for a moment what portion of health-care spending is due to physician fees. A study by Jackson Healthcare and reported in *Healthcare Finance News* (May 29, 2012) found that physician compensation in the United States is among the lowest of Western nations on a percent basis. This conclusion is based upon salary data from the Organization for Economic Co-operation and Development (OECD) and the Medical Group Management Association. Physicians' salaries comprised

8.6 percent of our nation's total health-care costs; among the comparable Western nations, only Sweden had a lower number, at 8.5 percent.

Comparison numbers for several countries are: Germany, 15 percent; Australia, 11.6 percent; France, 11 percent; United Kingdom, 10 percent; United States, 8.6 percent; and Sweden, 8.5 percent.

Other data taken from a response to an article in the *New York Times* "Week in Review" (July 29, 2012) made the point that physicians' pay is about 20 percent of the total national health spending. Of this total, however, half is absorbed by physicians' practice expenses, to include malpractice premiums but excluding the amortization of college and medical school debt. Thus, the net to the physician is about 10 percent. *Forbes Magazine* (April 3, 2013) published in its online site an opinion piece on rising health-care costs that put physicians' salaries at about 10 percent of health-care spending. This seems to be a rather constant number with a small range around it. It is clear that physicians' salaries are not a major driver of health-care costs. They do remain, however, a convenient scapegoat, real data notwithstanding, for politicians and insurance companies who never are slow to point to the physician as the cause of rising health-care costs in order to direct attention away from the real problems.

The more important causes of the disproportionately rising health-care costs were and are: administrative expenses, insurance premiums, technology, hospital costs, and chronic disease— much of it brought on by self-destructive lifestyles (smoking, drugs, alcohol, obesity, and a sedentary life). These all have a much greater impact on rising health-care costs. Yet even though physicians are a relatively small part of the cost of health care, they remain quite visible. The historic stance taken by organized medicine against broader access to medical care has played a role in this state of affairs. A similar intransigence to the acceptance of some paramedical personnel by many physicians' organization similarly put organized medicine or "traditional medicine" in a bad light.

Those of us new to medical practice in 1965 paid scant attention to these changes in the payment system, as there were internships and residencies to deal with. The familiar operational chain remained solidly in place: physician, nurse, and patient. Physician extenders were yet to make a significant appearance. There were technical personnel in hospitals and clinics, to be sure, but they provided ancillary services in laboratories and radiology and not direct patient care. Surgical technicians were new, and, by and large, registered nurses filled these positions.

Then there was the matter of Vietnam with its attendant conscription of men into military services. For those of us who became part of the military, a world opened where there would be a life-changing array of new experiences and considerations. Among these were physician extenders of many sorts (I use this term a bit loosely to make the point about the various forces that would come to bear on the delivery of medical care after that war): medical corpsmen who, though narrowly trained, were many times quite good at what they did and often took serious risks to do their jobs; technicians who performed a variety of tasks that simplified the work of physicians (some of these positions existed in civilian medicine, but not to the degree with which they were employed in the military); helicopter medevac pilots who greatly improved survival of the wounded and applied their skills to air ambulances back home. There are other examples, but these will serve.

One feature of the work of many of these people was overlooked: not only did they do procedures generally reserved for physicians in the civilian world (e.g., start intravenous fluids or blood infusions or do some surgery to avoid or mitigate larger surgery later), they also made the decisions to do so. The latter is a major distinction, and slowly it became clear that nonphysicians who had some training could make these decisions. This had its start with the corpsmen in World War II and then expanded rapidly in the Korean War, but it came into full flower in Vietnam.

In 1965, President Lyndon Johnson received a report titled "Accidental Death and Disability: The Neglected Disease of Modern Society." It showed that they were the most important causes of death in the first half of life. This report led, in 1969, to the first nationally standardized curriculum for the training of emergency medical technicians. They were largely confined to ambulance work. Shortly thereafter, this was expanded to create EMS-P (paramedics). The first residency program to train paramedics was established at the University of Cincinnati in 1972. The public gradually became aware of paramedics and what they could do, in part because of a popular television show *Emergency*. In 1979, advanced cardiac life support became widespread, and paramedics were certified in this in the mid-1980s. I was taught this as a medical student and used it many times in the hospital setting as a student, house officer, and faculty physician. But it took about twenty years for it to become a widely used, lifesaving technique applied by nonphysicians. In the early 1980s, the paramedic appeared in early studies with firefighters in Seattle, Miami, and Los Angeles, among other places, that showed that these people, using a rapid response system, could save lives.

Unlike the situations in the former wars, people who served in paramedical roles in Vietnam came back home to a social milieu that was looking for ways to lower costs and provide more care to more people who were underserved or ignored. These veterans—helicopter pilots, corpsmen, and surgical technicians—began to fit into medical care and alter its practice. With many skilled helicopter pilots suddenly available, helicopters began to be used in construction, transportation of people and goods, and delivery systems of many sorts. Among these was the transportation of injured or acutely ill people to medical facilities. The effect in the civilian world was the same as on the battlefield: lives were saved and morbidity lessened by decreasing the time to medical care.

Corpsmen, now being reinvented as paramedics, began to ride not only in ambulances but in helicopters as well, and medical care began at the site of injury. This expansion of the medical care delivery system—a direct result of the conscription of men into the Vietnam War—rapidly altered medical care delivery and the physician's role, and in a very beneficial way for patients. The unnoticed effect was the tacit and growing understanding that many acute medical problems could be addressed outside of hospitals and physicians' offices. In fact, waiting for the patient to be brought to a hospital for care by a physician could be deleterious.

It was recognized in the early 1970s that patients with the same types of acute illnesses might be managed better if they were grouped and cared for by a dedicated team with all the necessary equipment, therapeutic agents, and specially trained personnel in one place. Similarly, delegation of what heretofore were considered to be physician responsibilities could be assigned to nurses if they received additional training. This was the morphing of a military use of personnel (i.e., train the people to do what is needed at the site where it is needed). The cardiac care unit was born, and the general intensive care unit followed in short order. The birthing of these units was not simple; in many places the labor was long and the delivery difficult. History was very much against it, and their very existences made it clear that the magic of the physician could be taught to others, albeit at a technical level, yet with beneficial effects for the patient. Nurses were empowered to do diagnostic work, make decisions, and initiate therapy if needed. The physicians and nurses became a genuine team, and the linear relationship began to blur a bit.

In 1970, I was a ward medical resident at Barnes Hospital at Washington University in St. Louis when the cardiac care unit opened there. There had been much controversy about the unit, which had been championed by a young cardiologist on the staff. I did not know then, but realized later, that he had, in effect, put his academic career on the line when he did this. Many eyes were watching to see what would transpire: an expensive way to care for patients who historically had been kept in their own rooms or an efficient and better way to manage these dangerous illnesses. As luck would have it, I was the first ward medicine resident to be assigned to the cardiac care unit when it opened. That also meant that my impressions and judgments would influence the medical residents who would follow. I pride myself on having an open mind—some benighted might disagree—and was determined to give this experience a fair evaluation. It was not as though my thoughts would have any effect on the unit's future, or anyone really even cared what I thought about it, but I saw it as a node in the progression of cardiac care that could change how we did things and wished to judge it dispassionately.

It took less than two hours to realize that the unit was not an aberration in medical care but rather the model for the future. There were relatively few patients per nurse, and as a result, the nurses knew them very well. The patient–nurse rapport was excellent, and I soon learned that I could rely on not only the information given me but also the judgment that accompanied that information. Cardiac arrests, which were commonplace in such a unit, were managed instantly, efficiently, and smoothly, and sometimes they were anticipated by watching the cardiac rhythm on the monitor. From the point of view of teaching, it was even better. A month in that unit was an opportunity to experience every common cardiac disease or event many times; it also was a place where uncommon cardiac problems were sent and one experienced those as well. I was too new to medicine to grasp the full breadth or implications of what I was seeing—with respect to the changes technology would make in patient care or the many roles that nonphysician caregivers would play—but there was little doubt in my mind that the patient care model was undergoing a material change.

My time in the military gave me a grudging, and then wholehearted, appreciation of the skills and enthusiasm of corpsmen. Diagnosticians they were not, but they were doers and rather good at it. This was not novel, but it was to me and started a line of thought about medical care extension and a reexamination of my reference frame. The experience in the cardiac care unit did the same with respect to the efficient use of technology and what nurses and other paramedical personnel could do when given the opportunity. These experiences became useful several years later because they provided a background that would allow a more dispassionate assessment of the changes that were to take place in the delivery of medical care. They also produced some bias toward acceptance of these changes rather than a reactionary state of mind.

The military corpsmen who emerged from the Vietnam War were well trained and were looking for ways to put their skills to work. At the same time, in this country there was a serious shortage of primary care physicians. Dr. Eugene A. Stead, of Duke University, brought together four navy corpsmen in 1965 who would become the first graduating class of physician assistants (PAs) from Duke University in 1967. The term "PA" was coined by Dr. Stead. The concept actually was somewhat older. Dr. Amos Johns in the 1940s had trained unskilled assistants to provide rural medical care under his supervision. However, it was Dr. Stead who formalized and organized it and turned it into a profession.

Unlike nurse practitioners, who began to develop about this same time and for similar reasons, PAs had considerable training in the military as corpsmen and had been the first responders for many injured people. Nurse practitioners used a nursing training model, but Stead based the PA curriculum on the fast-track training of physicians during World War II. The average length of a PA education program is twenty-six months (three academic years). Applicants to PA programs must complete at least two years of college courses in basic science and behavioral science as prerequisites to PA school. The majority of PA programs have the following prerequisites: chemistry, physiology, anatomy, microbiology, and biology. Additionally, most PA programs require or prefer that applicants have prior health-care experience. The latter is more important now than at the onset since the PAs then had combat experience or clinical experience in forward hospitals. This is less true today, and they may be more academically qualified than they are clinically when they complete training. The extent of clinical training of the PA probably varies directly with US military activity abroad.

The PA concept gained federal acceptance relatively quickly, probably because of the nature of the training and the clinical experience acquired in the military. Realizing that this was a creative response to the shortage of physicians, the organized medical community supported the PA concept and aided in the setting of accreditation standards and a national certification process. As early as 1970, Kaiser Permanente became the first HMO to employ PAs. The following year, the American Medical Association recognized the PA as a profession.

Some years later, the early 1980s, I was chief of medicine at St. Louis City Hospital and needed to conserve and protect the time and energies of my medical residents. They could not manage seriously ill inpatients and a large outpatient clinic population without a decrease in the quality of care and exhausting themselves in the process. My response was to substitute physician extenders for residents. There were nurse practitioners available, but the times were such that they were not allowed to do much of anything. We put them to work anyway to staff the diabetic and hypertension clinics and retained a supervising medical resident in each clinic. The nurse practitioners freed about five medical house officers from each clinic to manage inpatients. The nurse practitioners were knowledgeable, anxious to prove themselves, and very popular with the patients since they spent more time with them than the house staff was able to do. It was a surprisingly popular solution for all concerned yet bitterly opposed by the senior medical staff.

Nurse practitioners (NPs) were a natural evolution from the nurse specialists who began to staff the various hospital intensive care units that developed after cardiac care units showed themselves to be valuable in the care of patients and efficient in the use of personnel, facilities, and equipment. The first NP program was developed as a master's degree curriculum, based on a nursing model, in 1965 by Drs. Loretta Ford and Henry Silver at the University of Colorado. It evolved in response to a nationwide shortage of health-care services at the time. Thereafter, a master's program for NPs was initiated at Boston College, and in 1968 a nurse practitioner program began in Boston. By 1973 there were more than sixty-five NP programs in the United States, and by 1980 there were over two hundred. In 1985, the American Academy of Nurse Practitioners was established and the discipline was formalized. It has since grown substantially. The first program at the University of Colorado was created from a group of public health nurses, and it specialized in pediatrics; other specialties were added as programs developed nationwide to provide primary care to underserved populations. The secretary of health, education, and welfare issued recommendations in 1971 that supported NP roles as primary care providers.

Thus, medical care expanded from the physician's office and hospital to outside clinics and to paramedical personnel who became the first responders that we know today. The use of paramedics, physician assistants, nurse practitioners, and other paramedical technical personnel unalterably changed medical practice. This diffusion of responsibility decreased the visibility of the physician and truncated the pedestal the physician occupied. These changes, instituted to provide good medical care in areas that were overused and understaffed, did much to correct the problems, and many people were better served. However, the care provided by these physician extenders is, of necessity, focused and of a technical level. Any evaluation of a patient in depth must wait until the physician is available. In the case of the paramedics, that takes place upon arrival in the emergency room; in the various intensive care units in a hospital, it occurs within that same unit and very quickly. When a PA or NP acting as a primary care provider sees a patient, the physician may not be involved at all. Under these circumstances patients receive care at a technical level, which frequently is adequate but sometimes is not. Many serious illnesses can present as a relatively simple array of signs and symptoms, and it takes some experience to ferret these out. In our system, only the physician has this experience. The quality of medical care is lessened under these circumstances even though the patient does not realize it. Yet it is considerably better than no access to care. In a medically underserved area, the PA and NP are quite valuable. In an urban area with available medical facilities, patients screened by physician extenders should be passed on to physician supervision quickly. Otherwise, quality of care deteriorates. This can be mitigated through a close and trusting interplay between the physician and the paramedical person. Under those circumstances this type of system operates at its best.

The last expansive change to the scope of our health-care system came with the enactment of the ACA in March 2010. The ACA, like Medicare before it, expanded the reimbursement system and made it more inclusive. These two financial bookends of our time period brought health care to many who could not afford it. The ACA was the other shoe that had waited almost fifty years after Medicare enactment to drop.

It was the great recession of 2008–2009 that acted as the catalyst for passage. Not only were about 20 percent of our people without medical insurance, but there also were many who had it and could ill afford it. The wealthiest country in the history of the world could not care for its own people. The ACA was ineptly crafted, it will cost much more than anticipated, and the rollout was poorly managed. Nevertheless, it has been a considerable benefit to many Americans. As of late spring of 2014, about twenty million people had gained health insurance under this act, and the uninsured dropped from about 18 to 20 percent to about 13 percent.

The provisions of the ACA that brought about this economic change were as follows:

- The guaranteed issue of insurance that prevents denial of coverage due to preexisting conditions.
- Health insurance policies that must meet minimum standards.
- The individual mandate that requires individuals not otherwise covered to secure a private insurance policy or pay a penalty.
- The certainty that low-income individuals will receive subsidies.
- The expansion of Medicaid eligibility.
- A mandate for businesses that employ fifty or more people to offer health insurance or pay a penalty. (This was delayed for a year since it was onerous for many businesses.)

This is a selected and edited list that bears only upon the inequities of health-care delivery (i.e., fee-for-service care based upon ability to pay). This was a major issue among the public until the enactment of Medicare and Medicaid and continued among the uninsured until the passage of the ACA. The bill is a major change in thinking for one of the most capitalist countries on earth and was bitterly fought. It was upheld by the US Supreme Court in June 2012 and clearly is the law of the land. It is far from perfect and will be changed several times before it is in its final form. Despite its flaws, it addressed an important social need that was widely perceived in the general population but largely ignored by the medical establishment.

The physician's influence and impact have been diluted in order to provide more and broader medical care. It began with the best of intentions, and most of those were realized: wider distribution of care for simple problems; care provided where little or none was available before; in some instances, a lower cost of care; and the sparing of physicians so their time could be used to better advantage. All of these benefits are undeniable. The sum has been broader access to primary care for the general population. Quality is assumed in the process whether it is there or not. The psychological cost to the physician is the interposition of people and policies between doctor and patient. The physician became the backup to the primary provider, and patients began to relate more directly to someone else.

THE ADVENT AND DOMINANCE OF TECHNOLOGY

ADVANCES IN SCIENCE TRANSFORM MEDICINE, AND THE PHYSICIAN BEGINS TO DISAPPEAR

THE EXPANSION OF THE HEALTH-CARE SYSTEM IN THE FORM OF physician extenders brought about substantial changes in the processes of medical practice. However, they did not change the nature of medical practice. The patient–physician nexus still was the focus. The technological revolution in medicine, concomitant with the expansion of health-care providers, not only would change the nature of medical practice but also would disrupt forever the personal physician–patient relationship and transform medicine into more of a technical exercise.

In the early part of the second half of the last century came the beginning of discussions about the use of automation to assist in medical diagnosis and data management. Automation was vaguely defined, and the applications to medical diagnosis were more of a miasma than focused applications. The concept of "cybernetics" was only a few years into the popular literature, and the concept of "feedback" to slow or speed a process was in its infancy. Much of the change in medicine and in the role of the physician in the second half of the last century was due to the rapid advances in basic and applied science and their applications to medicine through the explosive growth of technology.

Most of this was not even imagined in 1960. The structure of DNA had been proposed only in 1953 by Watson and Crick in the journal *Nature* and then elucidated in a series of four more papers in that same journal by these authors and their coinvestigators in that same year. Consider that the genetic code—which nucleic acid bases coded for which amino acid—was not even known then. Fifty years later, the entire human genome has been sequenced and we know which parts of that genome code for proteins. About twenty-one thousand genes (2 percent) of the genome are active in the coding of amino acids for proteins. In all, about 80 percent of the genome is biochemically active, as we understand it today, and the parts that are not coding for proteins are coding for transcription factors that regulate the genome from the time the organism is formed in the womb until life ends. The nongenome DNA is the choreographer for the genome, signaling it when to turn on or off and modifying its activity. This has been an astounding advance in the understanding of the human organism. The technological advances that made scientific understanding like this possible changed the character of medicine completely and irrevocably.

The result of this has been that medical science itself, rather than guiding the directions of research, as it did in earlier years, has been guided increasingly by molecular biology, biophysics, and biochemistry. Rather than searching from the disease to the cause, as was the case in the early part of the second half of the century, it was basic science that has informed medicine. Two of the more recent examples of this phenomenon are the development of pharmacogenomics and advances in neurosciences.

The sequencing of the human genome made possible many investigations into the genome and its function and created, among others, the discipline of pharmacogenomics. This is the identification of genes that create tumors or are related to the causation of other diseases. This information can be used to create therapeutic agents that can, through their actions on these genes, specifically treat these diseases. By extension, it now has become possible to treat only those persons whose genomic expression is responsible for a tumor and avoid the use of these toxic agents in persons who would not respond anyway. This also simplifies clinical trials of new drugs directed at specific metabolic or genomic function by limiting the persons in the trial to those with the relevant genomic structure. These trials can progress more quickly, with fewer patients and better statistics, and result in more rapid approval for the use of the drug.

The beginnings of this scientific and technological revolution began to appear in the late 1950s. The development of diagnostic processes done in laboratories or diagnostic centers ultimately would put instrumentation between the physician and patient or, at least, make testing systems an integral part of the diagnostic process. This interposition, as the technology grew stronger and increasingly versatile, would come to dominate the relationship. Although some technology was available before 1950, there was an increasing awareness of the possibilities in the early 1960s and the appearance of applications in the early 1970s. These applications grew rapidly due to the emergence of computers. The advent of the computer and the rapid development of its power to collect, analyze, correlate, and store data in an easily recoverable manner changed our entire society in the second half of the twentieth century. Medicine was one of the human activities caught up in the change brought about by computing power. Since medical care was a lucrative business for those who thought of it in that way, and the supply of customers (patients) was seemingly inexhaustible, and the payment systems were apparently endless as well, company after company rushed to develop diagnostic tools that made use of computing technology.

Over about twenty-five years, the immense growth in computing power predicted by Moore's Law affected medical technology, as it did most things in our society. Miniaturization became commonplace, and those smaller instruments did bigger and better things. Analytical methods produced more information with less sample volume and returned the information in hours or minutes. Imaging techniques produced pictures of the insides of people within minutes after the tests were done. The result was *Star Trek* medicine: the application of technical methods to a sick person to produce a diagnostic result in a short time. The magic of medicine devolved into the computer chip, and the physician increasingly ordered tests and waited along with the patient for the results. The physician was not in charge, and that was clear to the patient. The physician's skill was decreasingly what he carried in his head and increasingly in the array of diagnostic technology that was available.

This demand for and the push to provide diagnostic information rapidly outgrew departments of pathology in the 1950s that did clinical laboratory testing almost as a sideline. As the applications to diagnosis expanded, so did the need for specialists, and there was the realization that laboratory diagnosis was becoming a medical specialty of its own. The academic discipline of laboratory medicine was born. Physicians who were pathologists soon had to choose between anatomical and clinical pathology—that is, would you do autopsies and look at microscope slides as a career, or would you involve yourself in analysis of body fluids and the development of the technology to do so? The former had been a mainstay of medical and surgical diagnosis for more than a century; the latter was very new and held enormous promise. It required knowledge of medicine, an interest in analytic procedures and instrumentation, and an interest in economics and business. In a relatively short time, independent clinical laboratories began to appear to provide service to hospitals that were not large enough to support the increasing demand for and expansion of laboratory facilities. Ancillary services grew along with these laboratories: pickup and delivery of samples from hospitals; shipment of samples across states; the creation of schools to provide laboratory technicians; and the creation of doctoral-level scientists to develop newer and better analytic methods. The creature that made all of this possible was the computer, with its ability to do rapid analyses and its capacity to manage more and more data, store and retrieve it, and then send out reports automatically.

Concurrently, medical imaging techniques were being developed that would change body imaging as dramatically as autoanalyzers changed clinical laboratories. X-rays, the dominant imaging technology that gave departments of radiology and radiologists their names, were discovered by Wilhelm Roentgen in 1895 and had an immediate impact in medicine. X-rays saw inside living patients' bodies without the need to cut them open. New applications of X-rays increased physicians' abilities to see details and movement inside the body. From the 1920s, contrast media were used to outline surfaces of organs—the stomach and the colon were two organs where this technique was most popular. Those who had a barium enema would not soon forget the experience.

In the 1930s, sequential X-ray images of sections of the body were made in a technique called tomography that provided thick-section radiographs of the body that could be viewed in sequence to provide an approximation of three dimensions. Forty years later, Godfrey Hounsfield combined X-ray technique with computing power to create the first commercially viable computed tomography (CT) scanner that produced three-dimensional images of the brain. This EMI scanner was produced and marketed by the English Musical Instrument Company, the same company that produced the recordings of the Beatles. Allan Cormack of Tufts University worked out a similar process and developed the mathematics of radiographic scanning at about the same time, and the two shared the Nobel Prize in Medicine in 1979.

Clinical Laboratory Diagnosis

Laboratory diagnosis was where technology made its entrance into medicine. Through the 1950s, biological specimens were gathered from various body fluids and tissues and then processed by hand. The tests themselves had some error, generally maximized when done individually using hand pipetting or similar measuring techniques, and the results were slow to return to the clinician, requiring hours or days. The need for automation was clear not only for reasons of speed in obtaining results but also for reproducibility, minimization of both intra- and inter-test variation, and general quality control. Leonard Skeggs built the AutoAnalyzer in 1958 as a means of managing blood testing, and it could do one test a minute—a remarkable improvement in throughput. Hans Baruch, also in the 1950s, invented the "Robot Chemist," which was quite similar but was the first machine to give a digital printout of results. Developments in computers and robotics through the 1960s provided increasingly sophisticated instruments, and by the 1970s the sequential multiple analyzer could process twenty tests every twenty-four seconds.

One of the early people who saw the implications for clinical medicine was Dr. George Z. Williams, chief of clinical pathology, at the Clinical Center in the National Institutes of Health. Writing in the early 1960s and thereafter, Dr. Williams connected the government support of medicine (Medicare and Medicaid) and increased patient populations, and the beginnings of group practice, with the need for more rapid and accurate testing panels for patient diagnosis. He also foresaw that there would be a tendency for physicians to accept laboratory tests without question and subordinate clinical observation to the laboratory diagnosis. He became a spokesperson for the need to have a physician in charge of laboratory medicine centers in order to correlate laboratory information with clinical diagnosis. "Laboratory medicine" was a term that would become common and replace "clinical pathology" in the medical lexicon. There was a corresponding shift, over many years, as pathologists began to specialize in this discipline and forgo the more standard anatomical pathology practice. Ultimately, laboratory medicine became its own discipline and separated from its roots in departments of pathology.

These divisions of laboratory medicine were the facilitators of the entry of technology into medical diagnosis. They played a major role in improving the quality of laboratory testing through the continual monitoring of test results and advocating for higher quality and efficiency standards as new tests and devices appeared on the market. One of the unanticipated side effects of this push for quality and efficiency was conflict between laboratory medicine as a recognized specialty and the many small laboratories in departments of medicine and pediatrics that were managed by subspecialists. These subspecialty tests were used for a narrow spectrum of patients cared for by that subspecialty and generally were unavailable elsewhere, including divisions of laboratory medicine. In addition, they provided sources of income to these subspecialty divisions that were predictably reimbursable and unaffected by insurance monitoring of patient care costs. The audible arguments between laboratory medicine and the internal medicine subspecialty labs were structured as issues of quality control, reproducibility, quality of technical personnel, and timeliness of results. The real agenda in all of this was the income source that these labs represented for the medical subspecialties, and they were loath to give them up.

Certain subspecialties had endoscopes and other instruments that could be used for diagnosis and would generate significant charges; other subspecialties did not have these and often used their laboratories to do testing for diseases managed by that subspecialty and for the generation of funds. This was particularly true of endocrinology, rheumatology, and infectious disease divisions. In the long run, the small laboratories slowly disappeared through a prolonged rearguard action, and testing was brought wholly into organizations that provided laboratory diagnosis as a profession. These were divisions of laboratory medicine, in academic centers, or departments of pathology or central laboratories in nonacademic institutions, or outside contract clinical laboratories. Data that required days for delivery now were available in hours. The people required to generate the data and manage them were trained on a higher technical level, and the throughput was rapid. The systems were scalable, the revenue significant, and the margins high. Patients and practicing physicians were the beneficiaries since all the necessary quality control and efficient practices were easily maintained in these laboratory organizations and the resulting data were more reliable.

The noble intent of improving the quality of laboratory diagnosis and the resounding success of the effort also had the originally unintended effect of creating revenue centers. These, over time, became cash generators that remained relatively free of scrutiny by insurance companies that paid for patient care. As a consequence, they were lusted after by hospital administrators, finance managers, and department chairmen and were exploited fiercely. Thus came to medical centers the epithets "cost center" and "profit center"; these terms and the concepts they capture were quite foreign to those of us in medicine then. But we quickly came to understand their meanings and the nuances therein. No one wanted to be a cost center, but many times that was inherent in the subspecialty practiced. Profit centers were treated well by hospital administrations and academic leaders. Business had entered medicine under the cloak of these innocent-sounding descriptors.

IMAGING TECHNIQUES

As in laboratory medicine, the enabling force for the development and increasing sophistication of body imaging was computers. They made other body imaging machines possible. "Scanning" machines took readings of the body and used computers to turn the data into visual images. Magnetic resonance imaging (MRI) was developed in 1973. Positron emission tomography (PET) was developed in 1975. PET scanners tracked trace amounts of radiolabeled materials injected into the blood and could make visual images of those parts of the body that were functioning in response to some stimulus. This led to brain scanning that is used today for diagnosis and, increasingly, for sophisticated research on how the various parts of the brain collaborate to perform complex functions.

Imaging techniques, such as nuclear magnetic resonance and positron emission tomography, have emerged over a few decades as sophisticated and commonly used diagnostic tools. All of these have brought better diagnosis and treatment and have required trained technicians to manage them. The unanticipated consequence has been the marginalization of the practicing physician where he or she intersects those areas of medical diagnosis. The test and the technician have been inserted into the physician–patient relationship, and control of patient management transiently passes from the physician in the course of diagnosis. This loosens the physician–patient bond as both the physician and patient await the data from the technician. This is not necessarily a bad thing, since the data-gathering instruments are so powerful, but the patient sees the physician as somewhat sidelined by the diagnostic process.

Most of the conventionally used methods of imaging the various parts of the body generally use tomography. This refers to the creation of sections through the part of the body to be examined by a penetrating wave. The results are converted into a visual image that can be examined by the physician. The wave can be an X-ray (the first of these techniques and known as CT scans); radio-frequency waves (known as MRI scans); positron emission tomography (known as PET scans); and ultrasound transmission tomography (sonograms, which use sound waves for evaluating blood flow and the fetus in utero, among others). The manifold nontomographic uses of radioisotopes, which made their appearances in medicine about midcentury, certainly should be included. They began with the use of radioactive iodide to image the thyroid gland and then to ablate overactive thyroid tissue; there followed various scintigraphic (radioisotope) techniques to look at particular organs—the lungs, blood vessels, the vascular system, and others. These, although important, will not concern us here.

Our point is the effects on medicine from the translation of these concepts from physics into medicine. These and other methods of passing energy waves through a medium to examine differences in densities in the targets of those waves are used in disciplines as diverse as physics, oceanography, geology, and medicine, among others. The applications of some of these energy waves to medical diagnostics highlights how medicine has morphed from magic to mundane as computing revolutionized our increasingly sophisticated society and medicine along with it.

The applications of these techniques tended to consolidate themselves in departments of radiology. After all, the X-ray had been there for decades and the kinds of people interested perhaps more in diagnosis than in direct patient therapy were there as well. Nonphysicians with knowledge of physics began to gather in these departments as the potential of the applications of physics became clearer.

Currently, scanning machines are commonplace and provide information to physicians that can be gained no other way. They give us a look inside the body—everyone likes that—at the time the symptoms are present. In addition, PET scanning methods are allowing science and medicine to examine the brain as it works. This was an opportunity unimaginable until recent years. We have learned more in the past ten to fifteen years about brain function than in all of our history. This has come from the application of biophysics, through various scanning devices, to observe the brain as it receives stimuli and thinks. Thought processes can be traced through the brain as they move from place to place. The future of technology, primarily through biophysics, in the neurosciences is so broad and deep that the possibilities defy the imagination. With respect to current medicine, much of this will focus on converting the thinking process into a movement by a robotic extension. The short-term applications are directed toward allowing wounded veterans to bypass damaged limbs and spinal cords and mentally control mechanical limbs.

This already has been shown to be feasible and is beginning to be put into practice.

These advances in genomics and neurosciences require the focused energies of scientists and technicians just in their applications to medicine—a limited area when one considers the broad potential. They will move the physician further from the diagnostic and even therapeutic processes, but the benefits to patients appear limitless.

COMPUTERS

I was early in my career and happened to read an article that chronicled a study of interpretation of electrocardiograms read by cardiologists and by a computer. The two methods were shown to be about equally accurate. The conclusion in the article was that computers were no better than cardiologists. My conclusion was that the cardiologists were doing the best they could, but the computer was learning and would do better as time went on. I had no concept of just how much better the computers would do.

Several years later, when I was chief of medicine at a municipal hospital, the advance I expected became clear and very useful. We had a time-consuming and contentious issue: a medical resident was expected to read all the electrocardiograms (EKGs) for the hospital. This was supposedly a teaching exercise for the medical residents. It was not, since there was no supervising faculty member present. It was a billing exercise for the hospital. The solution came in the form of a new EKG machine that read the results itself. This eliminated any requirement for a resident to review the EKGs, and the hospital could still bill for the test. That eliminated all objections from the administration. The tracings were kept in patients' charts and remained available so the abnormal tracings could be used for teaching purposes. The time saved for the house staff was considerable. The senior staff opposed it, largely because it was a change, despite the fact that the outcome was positive for everyone. This is a small and personal example of the increasing uses and benefits of technology. The EKG is an exercise in pattern recognition most of the time (there are times when it is necessary to understand the electrical vectors involved), and pattern recognition is something at which technology excels.

I believe it is not possible to overstate the importance of computers in changing medicine—and indeed most of human activity—in the past fifty years. The unintended effect, for our purposes here, was to dilute further the role of the physician in medicine and diminish the physician–patient relationship. The enormous benefit was the multiplication of diagnostic power and creation of new methods for evaluating patients. Dr. Eric Topol, in his book *The Creative Destruction of Medicine*, has an interesting illustration that shows the appearance of various digital technologies from 1970 to date. The acceleration of the influence of technology in society has undergone a series of inflection points as cell phones, personal computers, the Internet, and various digital devices made their appearances. The growth of computing power due to the addition of digital methods and new instruments has been exponential. Computers had their effects on all of society, and their use in medicine and their effects on medicine are parallel to similar effects elsewhere throughout our civilization.

Our computerized armamentarium has improved medical diagnosis by making it more accurate and efficient. It has raised the cost of care concomitantly, very probably has decreased physician clinical acumen, and has made medical care a bit more like that in *Star Trek*—impersonal yet efficient and effective— and less like that provided by the beloved family doctor. Patients received more time, sympathy, and personal care from the latter, but who would go there again? These diagnostic and therapeutic improvements carried a price, and that price was in the cost to our national health-care economy and the weakening of the physician–patient relationship. The physician's arcane diagnostic knowledge gave way to technology based on science. We slowly became recipients of technical information and then were on the way to becoming skilled labor.

A concern that was voiced early in the use of new technology was the significant overuse and overreliance on these in lieu of clinical judgment. It also was used increasingly in defensive medicine and raised the cost of care not insignificantly. As these new methods became available, it became possible for a plaintiff's attorney to ask the question, "Did you make use of all the available technology in evaluating this patient?" Extra tests, frequently unnecessary for the diagnosis, were done in order to anticipate this question in case it was asked later. Defensive medicine of this sort, done largely for self-protection, is very expensive. Tort actions against physicians became a major legal industry and had an unwilling ally in advanced technology.

ADMINISTRATION
OF MEDICINE

Sometimes I wonder whether
the world is being run by smart
people who are putting us on, or
by imbeciles who really mean it.

—Laurence J. Peter, The Peter Principle

ANOTHER EVENT FROM MY EARLY YEARS WAS A CONVERSATION WITH some physicians about the management of hospitals. I wondered if physicians should not be managing hospitals themselves since they knew more about patient care. The response was that physicians could hire people to do this; the medical staff really ran the hospitals anyway. I thought this an odd response since actually we worked for the administrative organization. For years afterward, physicians who recognized this disconnect and went into administrative medicine were considered, quite unfairly, as simply unfit for practice and their real importance not credited. Where did that lead? Look around.

The transformation of the administration of health care appears to have come about the way so many major alterations do— slowly, while few people were paying attention. In midcentury, physicians dominated the hospital, and the administration was effectively an arm of the medical staff organization. Formally, the administration was in charge of the hospital, and managers occupied themselves with the operations of the hospital and walked carefully around the medical staff. Strong administrators were uncommon and often were discharged if there were conflicts with the medical staff. Yet some physicians recognized the importance of a close alliance of administration and medical staff and the importance of bringing medical experience directly into hospital administration.

In 1975, the American Academy of Medical Directors (AAMD) was founded to create a professional organization for this discipline. The primary focus of AAMD activities was to encourage physicians to assume more active roles in the leadership and management in the health-care industry and to help physicians acquire leadership and management skills through educational programs. In 1989, the name was changed to the American College of Physician Executives (ACPE), and that has since grown into a large educational organization that grants various diplomas and other forms of recognition to its members who complete educational programs. There are many physicians in administrative positions in health-care organizations who have trained with the ACPE, but they do not appear to have altered health-care administration in the way persons who trained in business have done. Current senior executives in health-care organizations are selected largely on the basis of their corporate experience.

The failure of the medical profession to contain costs and the gradual increase of health-care costs from about 10 percent of the GDP in the sixties to 12 percent in the late seventies and the large number of uninsured or underinsured persons who were not receiving care prompted the federal and state governments to look more closely at the business of medical care. Much of that focus was on physicians and their charges, since these were quite visible, and less on the management of health-care organizations. Not that the latter were ignored—far from it—but sorting out efficiencies and waste was considerably more difficult than ratcheting down Medicare and Medicaid reimbursements. Much of that scrutiny was misplaced since physician costs are only about 10 percent of the health-care bill;

much of the rest lies in technology costs and inefficiencies in the management of the system.

Gradually it became clear that continuing to decrease reimbursements to physicians would ultimately be counter-productive. Physicians and their practices are like other people and their businesses in that they have fixed and variable costs. These are covered by charges for diagnostic and therapeutic measures by physicians and by charges for goods or services by businesses. A decrease in payments to physicians or businesses for their efforts are compensated for by efficiencies where possible and a reduction in variable costs. Ultimately, variable costs can be cut no more, businesses go out of business through bankruptcy, and physicians stop seeing Medicare patients in order to turn their efforts toward patients who can pay for services directly or through insurance. This is done not out of dislike for Medicare patients or an intention to "rip off" the system but rather a desire to keep food on the table and educate their children. The calculus is quite straightforward and, when presented in this reductionist manner, should make it clear that economics are pretty much the same in all sectors of commerce. Medicine is no different in that regard. What is different is the regard for patients by physicians. Patients are not customers or clients to a physician, whatever they may be to an administrator.

Into this, in the early to mideighties, came two major events that would change medicine forever: first, payment according to diagnosis-related groups (DRGs), the linchpin of various payment changes to come from both the government and the insurance industry. The major tool to create savings that would come from this was to be the more efficient management of physicians and their methods of practice. The second change was the appearance of midlevel business management people who appeared with the promise of instituting efficient "business practices" that would lower the cost of care. The increasingly incestuous relationship between the insurance industry and business conglomerates that managed ever larger and increasingly voracious "health-care delivery" systems was the vehicle that slowly carried medicine out of its delusional world where the physician–patient relationship still was paramount and with patient care as the focus and hurled it into the arena where quarterly earnings increases were the only thing that seemed to matter. This altered forever the nature of medical care and made it health-care delivery. The physician became an employee of a system.

The advent of DRGs in the mideighties was the first formal attempt to discipline not only physicians but also the health-care organizations by instituting a fixed payment for a given illness. The lists of DRGs were long and detailed, and the reaction to imposition of these sanctions was, predictably, to game the system by designating patients in the more complex diagnosis groups in order to maximize payments. These situations raised serious ethical problems for many physicians who tried to "play it straight" and thereby were chastised by their department chairmen or hospital administrators. Payers immediately assumed that the system was being gamed and demanded substantiation of the diagnosis designator. The paperwork began to increase as physicians spent more time on patient or teaching rounds to be sure the charts were documented fully—not just accurately but also with the use of appropriate jargon that would forestall an audit. This had nothing to do with honesty but rather being certain that a medically untrained auditor would find all the appropriate terms when reviewing claims. This was an unfortunately necessary exercise on both sides: the physician being certain that his or her reputation was not besmirched by overeager auditors, and the payer organizations being certain that they were not paying inflated claims.

It was 1986 when DRGs appeared at our hospital and the sky began to darken. Raising fees for extra work was no longer permitted. In response, it was decided that if a patient was in an academic medical center, then, by definition, he or she had a complex problem and we were to bill accordingly. Hospital rounds were no longer just about patient care but also about spending time to be sure the chart reflected the weighty thinking and justified the top level of billing for the visit. I did this for a while and then realized that the flow of teaching rounds had been completely subverted by the documentation process. The chart had been well documented before, but now the quantity of words became as important as their quality. Consequently, I began to make two sets of rounds. The first was teaching and therapeutic rounds with students and house officers and fellows; the second set, done alone, was to do the additional notes and checking of forms to justify the billing. This, of course, took more time—it probably cost me an additional hour or more each day when on service—but it led to better teaching. As a physician in academic medicine, the pressures of time were not those of physicians in private practice, but they still led to longer days and a definite feeling of being disingenuous regarding the billing situation. I felt I could not justify billing at the highest level all the time and backed down the charges as patients recovered and heard about it more than once from those concerned with revenue flow.

There came one afternoon in the clinic when I was talking with an older clinician. He was visibly upset and finally looked at me and said, "Damn it, Joe, I am not a health-care provider. I am a doctor." We talked about that and the direction of things for a while, and then we both returned to providing health care.

As the cost of care became an increasingly visible issue, there was agitation to "do something about it." The practice model was essentially the same as it had been for hundreds of years, even though group practices had begun to deliver care with more efficiency. Within medicine, there was unrest because of the income disparities associated with the ability to pass a device of some type into the body and thereby garner significantly more income. This led to increasing numbers of physicians who migrated toward the more lucrative specialties and subspecialization within those. This was a particular issue within academic medicine, where some divisions tended to operate at a loss while others had comfortable profits and often did not care to share them.

The pressures to increase clinical revenue were significant on those specialties that did not have a financial gimmick (forgive the word, but it is appropriate in this context).

My own introduction to the increasing cost of care came many years earlier, as a medical resident. I wrote a prescription for a new antihypertensive medication for a lady in the clinic at a city hospital. It had been a few years since I had been an intern because of military service and graduate school interludes, and new medications had appeared that I wanted to try. She thanked me and went away. About an hour later, she reappeared and dropped the prescription on my desk with the comment "I can't afford this." This, of course, destroyed my plan of treatment and waved a large flag in my face. We reworked the plan using some older and quite generic medications that cost very little. I managed her for a long time using those generics since even though drugs had changed, physiology had not. It was the beginning of my slow, yet steady, appreciation of changing medical economics and the disparity of medical care in our society. At that time, it was beyond my comprehension how high the costs would go.

Partially as an attempt to simplify DRGs, which were not performing as well as had been hoped, and in a larger attempt to rein in costs, Medicare adopted the concept of relative value units (RVUs) as a reimbursement formula for physician services. Once again, the budget sword was directed at physicians and not (yet) at the health-care organizations. Prior to the institution of RVUs, physicians were paid a "usual, customary, and reasonable" rate for services; this led to variability in payment. In 1989, the Omnibus Budget Reconciliation Act established a Medicare payment formula for physicians using RVUs as a basis. For each service, a formula contains three RVUs: one for physician services (52 percent), one for practice expense (44 percent), and one for malpractice expense (4 percent). (Is there any other business plan that carries a line item designation for defense of lawsuits?) The three RVUs are multiplied by a geographically weighted value to account for variations across the country, and then that figure is multiplied by a Medicare conversion factor to obtain a final payment. Moreover, since each service (RVU) in the fee schedule is determined using what is termed a "resource-based relative value scale," knowledge of how to determine which of these procedural codes to use for billing is very important. The wrong RVU used to calculate an invoice can lead to underpayment or overpayment—the former leading to a deteriorating office practice and the latter to a very unpleasant audit by Medicare.

Medicare and almost all health maintenance organizations (HMOs) in the United States use the resource-based relative value scale. One can imagine the increase in staff of physicians' offices, hospital administrations, and the Medicare offices required to manage this amount of data. What was, and remains, a laudable attempt to standardize charges and hold down costs also created an enormous bureaucracy to manage it. The costs of this bureaucracy and the enforcement of the rules of the payment system have added a very significant overhead cost to health care. Another unintended consequence probably has been the decline in primary care physicians (PCPs). Since payment is determined by RVUs, and subspecialists' RVUs are reimbursed at a much higher rate (since they are more complicated diagnoses), there is a great financial incentive to leave, or not to enter into, primary care medicine. This has brought about the shortage of PCPs and the increasing use of NPs and PAs as PCP stand-ins. The attempt to control costs—which it certainly did not do—has led to a health-care system dominated by financial considerations. These attempts in the 1980s to manage costs brought about the large increase in health-care bureaucracy with its ever-increasing costs and a decline in the quality of primary care as these changes drove physicians away and sometimes required the substitution of PAs and NPs. As a society, we now have become accustomed to this decline and are about to have it institutionalized.

Variations on this type of payment scheme have been proposed, and payment for quality rather than for effort is one of them. This is a laudable goal, but there is the inevitable question of how to quantify this quality. Subjective scoring will not work since no one will believe it. Objective criteria, such as the use of algorithms in managing patients, are unsatisfying because they add more forms and people to move them about and simply indicate that appropriate boxes were checked during the care of a patient. This implies quality but certainly does not guarantee it. It actually can mask incompetence since it requires a much lower level of dedication or intellectual involvement in a patient's care to check off a form than to systematically evaluate a patient's signs and symptoms in the course of an interview and physical exam. Checking boxes on a form generally is a substitute for thought rather than something that will stimulate it.

As the eighties drew to a close, it was clear that DRGs, federal and state control of reimbursement, increasing involvement of insurance companies in evaluating and—God help us!—preapproving medical care, and a rapidly expanding bureaucracy to manage all this were generally making things worse. Administrators who had been brought into institutions to make things efficient had failed to do so. Largely they had expanded their fiefdoms and built a thriving middle management. Sorely needed administrative or organizational innovation essentially was nonexistent, while technology and the computer made advances almost on a monthly basis. The contrast between the technology of medicine and the management of medicine was stark. Medicine was functioning in a "high-tech" manner, while its management remained in a cottage industry format—and a bloated and obese format at that. Medical administrators, whatever their backgrounds, had failed completely.

Physicians were spending more time on forms and dancing with the various payment partners and inspectors and less time with patients. Patients were increasingly dissatisfied with the "medical experience" they received and were vocal about it. The physician was the point at which the patient actually touched the system, and blame tended to accrue to doctors since they were the only face that was a constant over a series of visits. The perception that much of a visit was involved with the bureaucracy of check-in and payment or with technological assessment did not enhance the professional image of the physician. This brought about calls for experienced businesspeople to manage a system that was seen to be spiraling out of control. Businesspeople were only too happy to offer their services.

FOR-PROFIT AND NONPROFIT

There is a Wall Street theory that
holds profits can be maximized
by minimizing the product.

—*Russell Baker*

Medicine lost its soul when big business entered into the management of health care. As corporate business practices made themselves felt, there was a fundamental shift in how medicine was practiced. Prior to this, the patient was the focus of the health-care system and the physician determined the nature of the interaction between the patient and that system. The physician was not the manager; he or she directed how the system performed relative to a given patient. Once corporate business practices began to drive health care, there was much advertising about quality, savings, efficiency, and improvement of care. However, the reality was that neither the patient nor the physician was a focus of the health-care system. Corporate earnings had taken first place.

This is not to decry the entrance of business practices into medical care. Their value has been recognized for centuries but only began to be seriously implemented about four decades ago as many hospitals that were nonprofit realized that good intentions were not enough. Most of these were associated with religions and had been organized for charitable purposes. There were notable exceptions, of course, but generally this was the case. In addition to managerial inefficiencies, university-affiliated hospitals also had large overhead costs over which they had little control. These were the extra costs associated with teaching of students and residents in training and the care of the medically indigent. These took a substantial part of the budget and generally were written off as teaching expenses. Administrators with business backgrounds began to replace administrators who had the best of intentions but not the fiscal vision to manage the institution through the changes that would occur. The manifestations of responses to these changes included the combining of hospitals; the amalgamation of specialties into one hospital; aligning groups of physicians on the staff of a given hospital in order to guarantee patient volume; the focusing of a hospital on a disease or small group of diseases; bulk purchase of supplies by groups of hospitals; and other standard business practices designed to cut expenses and raise revenues. Physician practices began to do similar things. Group practices were among the first changes, multispecialty groups appeared, single-specialty groups appeared, and practices organized around new technology (e.g., radiology, renal dialysis) appeared.

However, the focus of these hospitals remained substantially the same: the care of patients. Physicians had some sway over how business was conducted, especially in university-affiliated hospitals, and generally put patient care before fiscal issues. Administrators, by and large, also used good patient care as the goal and tried to put fiscal matters second to good medicine. This became increasingly difficult as new and disruptive technologies appeared, and in order to remain competitive it became necessary to acquire them and the necessary attendant personnel. The costs of technology, improved methods for doing various tasks, unreimbursed medical care (particularly in people who had no insurance and allowed a disease process to become extreme before appearing at the emergency room), coupled with demands by physicians for the new methods of diagnosis and treatment slowly pushed hospitals deeper into fiscal crises, and the demand for "better business practices" brought about the entry of corporate business into medical care.

This new corporate mentality contained a fundamental change that never was mentioned. It was lost in the giddy hyperbole about quality care at a lower price. The patient was, despite all publicity to the contrary, relegated to the status of a product. Publicity touted the number of patients seen and the costs to produce the product: a treated patient. (This is not the same thing as a patient well cared for.) Quarterly earnings became the focus of health care, and shareholders' returns and share price became the metric by which a hospital company was measured. The physician was no longer a confidant of the patient nor an advocate. The physician gradually became the manager who delivered the product. The value of the physician to the health-care operation was measured by the amount of product produced. The philistines had arrived in force, and the health-care system would not recover.

It was during the nineties that medicine fell increasingly under the sway of what were termed "corporate business practices." This led ultimately to our current situation where physicians who endeavored to remain independent organizationally now are rushing into the waiting arms of various health-care provider organizations. Alexander Pope's quote earlier on vice applies here with increased relevance. Each stage of the weakening of the physician–patient relationship came about slowly as physicians were required to increase patient visits per unit time; accept lower reimbursement for these visits; vie with insurance claims adjusters for compensation or the right to carry out diagnostic testing; immerse themselves in relative value arcana in order to maximize the earned reimbursement; and, in general, devote more and more time and psychic energy to defending the citadel of traditional medical practice against an onslaught of accountants, middle managers, directors, and executives. There never was an inflection point where one could say, "Stop! This isn't right. Look what is happening here." It was one directive at a time: a change in some administrative procedure; financial incentives to increase patient throughput; or fiscally oriented alterations intended to increase quarterly earnings. All these brought shareholder support and expanded executive perquisites. Individual practitioners or small group practices became increasingly less able to withstand the commercial pressure and sold their practices to local or regional for-profit health-care organizations to survive. In this process, the entrepreneur became an employee. We sold our patrimony to philistines because there simply was not a choice. The world does end with a whimper. Read *Animal Farm* again; it is a good summary of what was done and how.

Market forces now are an integral part of our health-care system. It was not the case in the mid-twentieth century, because physicians controlled the supply to a rather steady and growing demand. There was competition among hospitals in a region, to be sure, but neither physicians nor hospitals were plentiful. Physicians were sought after to bring patients to a given hospital. By the 1980s, the supply of physicians had increased and the number of hospitals had as well. Paramedical personnel were beginning to play a larger role, but the system had not changed substantively. In the 1990s, as businesspeople entered into the management of what was now health care, the system began to change both rapidly and radically. It grew to the point that it was about 14 percent of our GDP and had layers of management that were not there before. Nurses were playing a larger role, and physician assistants were becoming commonplace as it became apparent that by pushing caregiving down a level there were cost savings to the hospital. Technology also was rapidly becoming a major force and was used increasingly since the profit margin was large. Now, health expenditures amount to about 18 percent of the US GDP and 10 percent of the world's GDP. The global health-care industry turns over more than $6.6 trillion annually. Not only are market forces driving the health-care system, the health-care system itself, because of its size, has created market forces that did not exist twenty years ago.

This situation is the result of the application of corporate business practices to a service industry that never was intended to be managed in this way. Health care never had a product before; it cured or helped people who were diseased or injured. There were costs associated with that, and they were considered part of the price of having a civilization. As money played an increasing role in health care, it corrupted all that it touched: administrators sought more growth and better margins; physicians entered into subspecialties that provided greater remuneration; technology, device, and supply companies saw voracious markets for their products; and an educational system developed new courses and degrees to meet the demands for health-care personnel. As corporate people began to take over, the system was modified to fit corporate business models—a not surprising development. A treated patient became a product produced by the health-care industry. The well-being of that patient was honored more by lip service than concern. Persons who provided the services that produced this product became workers in an industry and were managed accordingly. The people who bought the product—insurers of various sorts—were billed for it. The captains and officers of the industry were compensated as if each product turned a profit and were rewarded handsomely. Shareholders who bought equity in the health-care industry expected, and generally received, consistently increasing quarterly earnings. They, in turn, acquiesced in the large rewards given to upper management. Insurance executives were correspondingly well treated since a growing population that bought more policies increased the bottom line of insurers. The stage was set in the midnineties for an unholy alliance between insurance companies and the executive management of for-profit health-care companies. The alliance was adversarial, since the health-care organizations tried to game the insurers and the latter responded by choking off payment for services when possible and raising premiums. In this joust, physicians and caregivers simply were the horses that the two managements rode.

The fact that there actually is no profit to the health-care system as a whole, in the usual sense of that word, is understood but has not been noised about. It does not make a product; it provides a service. The value it adds to what it terms a product, the patient, is intangible to the system. A patient discharged from a hospital represents an expense. The bill for this expense is passed to an insurer. When it is paid, there is a credit back to the hospital, and what, thus far, has been an expense to the hospital now represents a real profit because of the markup. The insurer does not gain from paying for (buying) the product; it also is purely an expense to the insurer. Consider: If I have a construction company and buy earthmoving equipment, there is a profit to the manufacturer both because of the value added to the steel, which has become a machine, and the markup to me. There is a profit to me as well, since the machines add asset value to my company, and I profit by using them to do more construction. That is a good business transaction for buyer and seller.

Health care is different. Unlike my construction company, there is no value added to the insurer from the products (patients) paid for. They are pure expense. The only way the payer can continue to buy the products from the hospital is if young, healthy people who do not need the insurer's product (a health insurance policy) continue to buy it. The insurer's profit comes from unused inventory—money. The nature of health care intrinsically does not lend itself to large profits. What we are seeing now is unbridled capitalism (i.e., greed) driving a system that cannot last.

The hospital provides a service that costs it money. The insurance company pays the hospital. People who fear disease and its consequences buy insurance. It is a cycle—a sequence of expenses marked up and shifted progressively around the cycle.

Without a steady stream of insurance policies and new people to pay for the increased expenses of the old, the system fails.

This always has been the case in the insurance business, but it is coming to a head now with the implementation of the ACA. Surprisingly, people who do not need the product (health insurance) are not buying it; people who think they do need the product are buying it. Who would ever have imagined that this might happen? The inevitable result will be that recalcitrant customers will be compelled, in one way or another, to buy insurance and the policy costs will go up for them and everyone else as well. Once an industry becomes artificially large and a major part of the GDP, there is much profit to be made, but it is on a shaky foundation. There are only so many healthy people around to support the growing number of older and less healthy consumers. This is likely to change, in the short term, as younger people realize the importance of health care for catastrophic illness and begin to purchase insurance, as appears to be happening now. In the longer run, however, there will be increasing numbers of retired baby boomers and not enough younger people to sustain the health-care system as we know it.

Health care represents an expense—a cost center—for all concerned: the person with the illness, the hospital that manages it, and the insurer who pays for it. The value added to the product is realized only by the patient and is intangible—he or she feels better. The demand for the product (health) starts with the patient. The hospital fills the need, marks up the cost unconscionably, and passes it to the insurer. The insurer contests the cost, pays as little as possible, and, if possible, raises the premiums on the patient. If that patient has a chronic disease or is older and beginning to wear out, then the value added to the patient from health care decreases while the demand from that same person increases. This is fundamentally different from the usual business: when the product declines in value or the costs to produce it become excessive, the business cancels production or goes out of business. That is why medicine never was intended to be a business. If one applies corporate business practices to medicine and expects to continue to generate a profit, rationing of care will be inevitable.

How will the rationing be done? First, as is currently in progress, is to have more people seen by personnel with less training. Primary care physicians will morph into nurse practitioners and physician assistants. Take the physicians out of the equation as much as possible. They cost more, and they make noise if you squeeze them too much. A lower level of care costs the hospital less, and the throughput is greater. It is a perfect business model—lower quality and more of it. The trick is to convince patients that things are just fine, and that is done by advertising the cost savings. Recently I saw a sign outside a grocery store, one of the large chain stores with a small clinic inside. It read, "Sports physical, $33.00 and get 50 added gas points." Who could resist that? The store management is playing the odds, and quite cynically. Most adolescents who play sports are quite healthy. The chance of missing something important is small; the chance of being sued for this is smaller still. The parents believe that their child received a high-quality exam, somehow mentally equating a physician-quality exam with a grocery store clinic. We are being told that low quality is perfectly adequate, and look at the money you save.

How else will rationing be done? This is where it gets sticky. At some point, Grandma will become a burden on society, both to our society at large and to the family society from which she came. We are encouraged to have end-of-life guidelines—something with which I agree—since they ease decision making for a family. They also save money. The baby boomers are moving into the golden years and bringing with them a variety of chronic illnesses. Because of the large number of people retiring and the smaller number of persons paying for the running of the country and its excesses, there will be awkward questions raised during the next decade. The rationing of life is inevitable; it will become only a matter of how to sell it to the public.

There is tension within the system since costs are exorbitant and cannot be passed on easily to insurers. The physician as an employee of the system is squeezed by management to increase productivity and forced to spend less time per patient and thereby increase throughput. The use of procedures and tests is encouraged since these are readily marked up and passed on to payers. The difficult-to-control variable is the physician–patient interaction, the event of most interest to both participants. Physicians who still are in individual or group practices do not have the squeeze from management—at least not to the same degree—but deal almost constantly with insurance reviewers whose job it is to question diagnoses and physician services. The inevitable consequence is the absurd situation, which now is commonplace, where insurers decide what sorts of treatment patients receive through the simple expedient of withholding payment for services they will not approve. Physicians are put into the position of practicing medicine with the insurance company in mind rather than focusing completely on the well-being of the patient.

Sachin Shah, a physician affiliated with Doctors for America, quoted in a *Forbes* article (*Pharma and Healthcare* article [February 12, 2014]), points to the enormous profits associated with the medical insurance industry: "The five largest health insurance companies—WellPoint, United Health, Aetna, Humana, and Cigna ... earned over $3.3 billion in profits [between April and June 2011]." He also contends that "profit in the health insurance industry is the single greatest barrier to building an efficient, sustainable system of healthcare in this country." I certainly agree with that statement, and most physicians would as well. Insurance companies monitor the physicians' activities closely, and physicians frequently are required to justify treatment of a patient to an insurance adjuster before beginning therapy. This is practicing medicine without a license on the part of the company adjuster and is unconscionable but now is engrained into the health-care system.

Peter Ubel, the author of the article in *Forbes* mentioned above, also makes an important distinction: that of profits and income. His point—with which I agree but about which I also have some reservations—is that the basic issue is greed. That is certainly true. Profits are funds left over after all expenses, deductions, and taxes are taken out. Some major expenses are the salaries paid to health-care executives and never appear in the profits; they are expenses. Mr. Ubel also makes the valid point that the health-care system could be fully nonprofit yet still have high costs since executives are rewarded handsomely, even those in nonprofits. He points out that the CEO of the Mayo Clinic earns about $2 million a year; the CEO of Blue Cross/Blue Shield of Illinois made $16 million in 2012. If these are used as markers for salaries throughout their health-care organizations, the amount of money spent on salaries—especially when there is a large middle management group—is enormous. Add to that the costs of high-technology equipment and medical devices generally, and the people needed to run this equipment, and then the costs to provide health care become huge; all of this is listed on the profit and loss statement under expense. It never sees the light of day when profits are reported. If physician salaries are broken out of this, they actually are a miniscule part of the expense structure—some estimates are about 1 percent.

Here is a small but illustrative example: Several months ago I went to an emergency room because of painless swelling in the left leg. In an older person, in the absence of trauma to the leg, this conjures up a number of diagnostic possibilities, none of them good. The entire process was smooth and rapid. It was door to door in one hour. Blood was drawn, two radiographic tests were run (about twenty minutes), no deep vein clots were found, and blood tests for clotting were negative. I was sent home with advice to watch this and return if the swelling did not decrease. There was no diagnosis made, although everyone agreed that the leg definitely was significantly swollen. This sometimes happens; we just do not know what is wrong. I did not send for a lawyer.

Over the next three days the swelling went away. Not long after, the bill arrived; it was $7,007. It is a rather large bill for one hour but perfectly consistent with current medical charges—which does not justify the cost, by the way.

This is how the charges were distributed: blood tests, $2,176; radiographic tests, $2,524; and ER usage (all costs), $2,307. The ER usage was 31 percent of the total; the laboratory and technology costs were 69 percent. This is not an indictment of technology since it was essential in the evaluation. However, two blood tests—both done by an autoanalyzer at a cost of a few dollars, if that—I believe were not necessary and played no role in the diagnosis. Those two cost $1,191, or 55 percent of the total blood test costs. The ER costs included the physician's fee of about $225, or 10 percent of the ER cost and 3 percent of the total bill. All the rest in the ER usage was for PAs, nurses, some materials, and the use of the room. Physician fees are not driving the cost of medical care.

Any organization must manage its bottom line, whether it is an enormous health-care company, a large financial institution, or a small business; however, the greed generally associated with both of the former, in the form of absurd salaries, bonuses, and benefits—which are buried in the expense side of the ledger—constitute a significant percent of the costs of health care and are part of the reason for the exorbitant billings of health-care organizations, large financial institutions, and large legal offices as well. Mr. Ubel is correct: greed is the problem here. The greed is found throughout the bloated middle management ranks and the higher-level executives in the health-care companies; it also is found in these same ranks of the large corporations that supply drugs, devices, and computer-driven technology to health-care companies. Wall Street recognized this many years ago: health-care sector companies have been desirable stocks to own for more than two decades.

However, I must disagree on one point with Mr. Ubel, or alter the emphasis, at least. The pressure on for-profit organizations to increase the profit margin is greater than in nonprofits. He concedes the point in his article. This pressure for quarterly earnings increases requires for-profits, since they are not decreasing the salaries of those who manage them, to continue to raise prices in order to keep the quarterly earnings growing. The nonprofit organizations have much less pressure to do this. They must have a profit margin to put back into the business in order to make it grow and manage inflationary costs, but the quarterly earnings pressure is not the same. Let us look at the two systems. This is relevant to our examination of what has transpired in the lives of physicians since they now are increasingly beholden to institutions and, as a group, are not a force in the direction medicine is taking nor have they been over the past twenty years. Physicians are tarred with the brush used on health care even though they have virtually no influence over it.

There are three types of health-care organizations: for-profit, nonprofit, and governmental. The latter is the caregiver of last resort and may be considered as a variation of nonprofit; however, it is not relevant to our comparison. It is the first two that matter here. The distinction between these is important to the realities of health care today. It lies largely in the pressure created by investors and upper management to show increasing quarterly earnings. In terms of function, the two types of institutions are quite similar in the care provided, and the patient mix is similar as well. It has been shown, however, that for-profits tend to have a greater concentration of high-margin procedures than nonprofits. For example, for-profit hospitals are more likely to offer procedures that have a higher profitability, such as cardiac surgery. Moreover, as described by Jill Horwitz, a law professor who has done much research in this area, for-profits respond more quickly to changes in financial incentives. When services become more profitable—home health care, for example—the likelihood of for-profit hospitals to offer the services more than tripled. These hospitals dropped this care when a change in the law made it less profitable. Nonprofits went through a similar change, but it wasn't as fast or dramatic. For-profit hospitals also are more responsive to financial incentives than nonprofits, both with respect to their decisions to offer services and in their willingness to operate at all. Under financial pressure, for-profit hospitals are more likely to close or restructure than nonprofits.

In addition, their upper managements are paid considerably more. A study in the *Journal of Law, Economics, & Organization* found that the total monetary compensation for the two top executive jobs was significantly higher in for-profits, and the composition of that compensation (base salary and bonuses) differed as well. Bonuses were both absolutely and relatively greater in the for-profit organizations. In particular, there were greater rewards for performance that could be more easily measured. One of these, of course, is a profitability target. Meet that target and bonus is paid; there is considerable effort given to meeting that target and lesser targets as well, since they also generally are linked to performance and, hence, bonus. There is the major influence of the requirement of for-profits to generate a profit that can be returned to shareholders and also to manage the business in such a way as to maintain or increase the price per share of their stock. This is an important driver of upper management in any for-profit organization, and health care is no exception. None of this has anything to do with the delivery of health care. The patients in either for-profit or nonprofit hospitals have essentially the same caregiving experience. The difference has to do with the care and feeding of the management of the two systems.

Another difference appears to lie in the types of people found in each institution. The best of the nonprofits may have base salary structures similar to those of for-profit; however, there are no stock options since usually there is no stock. The bonus structure often is not there or is less important since there are no profitability targets to reach. Management and employees of nonprofits, in lieu of stock options and bonuses, often receive attractive benefits packages that may include vacation time, tuition reimbursement, retirement packages, flexible work schedules, and nonqualified deferred compensation programs where there may be no limits to contributions. There are other variations on benefit packages. A major benefit is time. Not uncommonly, it is a shorter or lessened workweek that can be used for personal time of the person's choosing. This is an intangible, but strong, incentive since the major problem with working all of one's life is the loss of time when one's family is young and developing.

Historically, health care has been medical care (i.e., places where physicians provided treatment for acute and chronic disease), and it was not for profit. These institutions were termed "charitable" and existed to serve the community. They began largely as hospitals affiliated with religious groups—as far back as the Middle Ages—and as manifestations of the moral and ethical imperatives for humans to care for one another. The Hotel Dieu, in Paris, is considered to be the first of these and was founded in the year 661. However, the laws of economics have operated in the same ways forever, and the Hotel Dieu was bothered by cash flow problems from its inception. In 1505, a council of laymen and government officials was convened to manage not only the hospital but to organize what was essentially a network of medical care facilities and a plan to manage them. In addition, even in the early years of the Hotel Dieu, distinguished clinicians who worked there had offices nearby, and specialty hospitals sprang up as well. Thus, the for-profit hospital industry had its beginnings not long after the first nonprofit hospital appeared. This ethos that brought the Hotel Dieu into being still was present even in the mid-twentieth century. By and large, hospitals were nonprofit, and most had religious affiliations.

Academic institutions, beginning before midcentury, often had religious or municipal hospitals affiliated with their medical schools. These latter hospitals were the results of regional and federal governments recognizing an ethical requirement to care for citizens in need. The affiliations with academic centers were mutually beneficial since the academic centers used these facilities for training, and, in turn, some of the costs of care were shifted from the municipal governments to the academic centers. When for-profit hospitals began to proliferate in the 1970s, the ethical implications became immediately apparent. The arguments ranged then, exactly as they do now: "Competition in the delivery of health care will create a more effective and efficient system" versus "The pursuit of profit is antithetical to the values of medicine and will decrease access to medical care for the impoverished." Crudely restated: you can make money or do the right thing. It is not quite that simple, but almost. It also is clear which side of that balance had more weight.

It was evident from the beginning that for-profit institutions decrease the access to health care for patients who cannot pay. This is done by demanding evidence of ability to pay before admission or treatment. This requirement changes the payer mix of that hospital toward the insured; the uninsured are discouraged from coming or are sent away. For-profit hospitals thereby can generate more revenues that allow them to expand into areas that are convenient to paying patients. This, of course, expands revenues further and also, for reasons of geography and finance, takes them further away from nonpaying patients. As unpalatable as this may be from an ethical perspective, one can justify it in terms of economics. That is to say, "We are a business dealing in health care, we are not simply providing health care to people who need it. Those who need it and cannot pay should go elsewhere." However, when for-profits refuse to serve acutely ill nonpaying patients, it is a scandal that mocks us as an advanced civilization. Turning away acutely ill persons or trauma victims because they cannot pay should be illegal; moral suasion is ineffective. Episodes of refusal of emergency care are quite well documented; they are justified by a medical determination that the person is stable enough to be taken to a nearby governmental institution (your local municipal hospital).

Historically, nonprofits have used paying patients to subsidize nonpaying patients. This cost shifting also can be argued as unethical since it is a tax on those who can pay. The counter to that is those patients are paying the agreed price, and those who cannot pay are given a discount or written off. One may argue, but it clearly is a more humane approach to health care than denial of treatment. The rise of the insurance industry has benefitted the nonprofits by increasing coverage of their patient mix. Many large nonprofits also provide their own insurance programs and thereby help support the organization. This is another distinction between the nonprofits and for-profits, since the latter generally deal with outside insurance companies. However, this is beginning to change as the economic gain of bringing insurance in-house becomes more obvious. One glaring difficulty in all this is that municipal hospitals are left to take up the care of those who cannot pay. Unfortunately, they are disappearing since they are too expensive to maintain. This leaves those who cannot afford insurance outside the health-care system, and this is where the government is supposed to step in to help its citizens. The government's ACA legislation recently did that with mixed but generally positive results.

These inequities are particularly felt, not surprisingly, among those with lower incomes. This was documented, in part, in a Commonwealth Fund survey in 2013 of adults in eleven high-income countries. We rank last when financial access to care is considered. The respondents to the survey did not visit physicians; did not fill prescriptions; did not get tests or receive treatment that had been recommended; or return for follow-up care because of cost. The emphasis on payment up front, high deductibles, and the demands of corporate medicine have brought us to this. We really do not feel obliged to care for one another. There is some promise that the ACA will address this inequity as its provisions began to be felt. Unfortunately, there are twenty-three states that did not expand coverage under Medicaid programs, and this will leave many lower-income people without health insurance coverage. Time will tell how long it will take for the pressure of public opinion to change the payment hurdle and to move toward universal coverage.

There is one other change common to both for-profit and nonprofit health care that already is in play. That is, of course, the elimination of the physician as completely as is practical yet still maintaining the health-care business. Physicians cost more, they ask awkward questions of administrators and then wait for the answers, they make embarrassing observations regarding inefficiencies and illogical practices, and they are concerned about patients and do not like to push them through an office exam in order to satisfy administrative dictates. There is little doubt that if health-care organizations could eliminate physicians from the mix, they would do so as quickly as possible. The storefront clinics staffed by paramedical personnel are ubiquitous; the use of physician extenders in hospitals is the same. The obvious business model is to combine these and do all primary care with physician extenders. Relegate physicians to the second line of evaluation and have them see the patients that the first line was unsure of. The cost savings would be substantial since there would not be as many physicians needed, and the cost to the patient would not change. More testing technology would be used because the diagnostic acumen of the physician would not be there. The profit in testing would increase. The quality of care would drop, but, as I pointed out earlier, most people would not know. There are those who see this as entrepreneurship at its best: higher throughput, lower costs, and larger profits. Quality would remain an intangible that never is measured but would be bruited about since it can be equated with throughput. Patients will bear the burden of this. The terrible thing is that younger people entering the medical care system will not know what they have lost because they never will have seen it.

There is another potential issue associated with this, and that is misdiagnosis. It is directly related to the short time of the physician–patient interview, will be exacerbated as physician extenders assume the role of the primary care physician, and will be reflected in the increasing costs of defensive medicine and malpractice litigation.

As long as there are humans, there will be human error. However, we all try to minimize it, especially in medicine, where human suffering or death may be the result. A study by Singh, reported in the *Wall Street Journal* (August 8, 2014, pg. A11) and published in *BMJ Quality and Safety* describes the problem. He and his colleagues reviewed diagnostic data on the entire US adult population and concluded that about 5 percent are misdiagnosed. One can argue that this is a very good record—95 percent correct—but it still leaves twelve million people misdiagnosed each year. The issue is large. The Institute of Medicine is studying it as well, and will issue a report in 2015. Singh recommended some steps to reduce the problem.

The first is to improve communication between physicians and patients. Every medical student knows that the patient will tell you the diagnosis if you simply sit and talk long enough to achieve good communication. The business approach of "patients per hour" guarantees that this will not happen; it also guarantees that this 5 percent misdiagnosis is the minimum and probably will increase as patient interaction times are shortened or as less well-qualified persons are used to screen patients. Singh also makes the point, known by every practicing physician, that the time pressures and paperwork regarding reimbursement preclude spending more time with patients. Moreover, extra hours used to pursue a diagnosis (i.e., thinking or reading or researching) are not compensated and are discouraged by management through the use of metrics to measure throughput of patients. Correct diagnosis and treatment are not measured.

He also supported the use of electronic medical records for rapid information transfer and cross-checking of information. These will undoubtedly improve the situation, but it is the initial physician–patient interaction that is the critical point. If misdiagnosis increases as a result of business pressures to "produce," and less qualified people are used too much, then misdiagnosis will increase.

There are many who believe that a society as wealthy as ours has a moral obligation to care for all its members. Everyone in this country should have access to medical care. Unfortunately, that moral imperative left the building sometime in the late 1980s or early 1990s. There is an additional argument that for-profit institutions benefit from government-subsidized research and medical education. They benefit from Medicare and Medicaid as well, and, therefore, should contribute something to the commonweal. That there may be such an obligation never has been acknowledged by the for-profit industry except for a small budget allowance for some charity care that is written off. It, however, pales beside the write-offs for overcharges for laboratory tests billed to Medicare.

Where is the physician in all of this? The physician is not a player in these systems except within institutions where he or she sits on various planning and review committees to make recommendations or on internal review groups to assure quality of care. These are important functions, but they do not rise to the level of managing the institutions or the direction of movement for the health-care industry. It is this exclusion from participation in upper management that has been such a frustration to physicians. They see the direction of movement, they see the problems and injustices, they experience the resentment of the populace, and they are targeted with much of the blame. They can do nothing about it; the system is beyond repair unless the profit motive is removed.

DEFENSIVE MEDICINE

DEFENSIVE MEDICINE IS A METHOD OF PRACTICE THAT DESTROYS THE SPIRIT AND IDEALS OF THE CONSCIENTIOUS PHYSICIAN

ANY DISCUSSION OF THE CURRENT STATE OF MEDICINE AND THE changes wrought on physicians over the past half century would be incomplete without some mention of the costs of physician self-defense. Some of these costs are significant and are measurable in terms of money. But there are other costs of defensive medicine that are intangible and probably more important. These are the effects on the physician and on the physician–patient relationship when a patient is viewed not as someone in need but as a potential litigant. The psychological effects of the predatory liability environment on the physician are enormous. Patients are more assertive, partially because of the advertising about seeking redress for real or imagined malpractice. There are more administrative burdens placed on physicians that consume time that must be taken from patient visits. Malpractice insurance premiums continue to rise, and the risk of being dropped by an insurance company should there be a lawsuit is always present. Add to this the continual background noise of television ads by law firms poised to step in and deliver monetary justice to the aggrieved patient. The final insult is that a malpractice judgment against a physician, regardless of its merit, will follow that physician forever.

This is all made more intense by the demands of health-care delivery systems—that physician employees see an increasing number of patients per unit of time. A major factor in avoiding lawsuits is the time that a physician and patient spend together (i.e., time spent building a personal bond). The time demands of health-care delivery organizations—both profit and nonprofit—militate against the formation of a bond that was the norm in the early part of the second half of the twentieth century. The aggregate psychological stress of these outside pressures of throughput and administrative burdens tends to push physicians into a defensive mode when actual liability risk alone might not do so. The destabilizing result of all this stress, unseen by the general public and ignored by corporate management, is the terrible discomposing effect on the psychological well-being of the physician. He or she is being forced to practice medicine in a way that not only is antithetical to the very nature of the person who became a physician but also to everything that person was taught in medical school and in subsequent training. Instead of being the advocate of and seeking the best for a patient, the physician is forced by fear of legal action and the pressure of fiscal demands not only to care for the patient but, concurrently, to defend against second-guessing by others. The result is defensive medicine, a method of practice that destroys the spirit and ideals of the conscientious physician. This is the true cost of defensive medicine; it is not the money.

The initial concept of litigation for medical malpractice was legitimate. Occasionally, people are damaged through negligence or accident; sometimes people are damaged through no one's fault. Unlike almost any other form of endeavor, people's lives and well-being may be placed directly in the hands of the physician in medical or surgical procedures. These kinds of high stakes are part of medical care. Sometimes people cannot be saved from the acute affliction they have. This is not medicine; this is life. Nevertheless, when there is a reasonable question about the competence with which a procedure was performed or whether a diagnosis was pursued appropriately, one can reasonably ask for recompense for damage inflicted. This is a perfectly legitimate application of personal injury law.

However, it also is clear that attorneys recognized this situation very early as a gift; the term "ambulance chaser" has been around for much longer than I have been involved with medicine. As the size of the GDP provided by health care grew over the past half century, the potential profit from medical malpractice lawsuits grew correspondingly. It is now, and has been for the past two or three decades, a very lucrative business. A glance at the ads on television sponsored by law firms that stand ready to be certain that your rights are respected and the implication that this can be equated to some dollar figure of recompense is quite good evidence of the lucrative nature of this business. This increase in litigation is not because there is an increasing amount of malpractice. Rather it lies in the recognition of the nuisance value of a malpractice suit. The time lost, serious mental anguish, distraction from professional obligations, the high cost of defending oneself, and the damage done to one's professional reputation are enough to deter most physicians from fighting even a frivolous suit. Although the physician may be innocent of wrongdoing, it becomes simpler to swallow one's pride and pay off the litigant rather than fight something through the courts. The litigant's attorney will take a percentage of the award and go off to sue another day. The physician's insurance costs go up, and overall malpractice insurance premiums ratchet up and continue to increment the cost of health-care delivery.

The law is what separates us from the Middle Ages. It is a monument to all that humanity aspires to be. Without it, property is not protected; what we consider basic human rights would not even exist; representative governments could not be maintained; and orderly economies would not exist. Without the law, there is no civilization. It is not science and technology that enable our global civilization and economy; it is the rule of law. For this reason, we have agencies to enforce the law and courts to adjudicate disputes. These mechanisms of redress reinforce the fact that we are a civilization that has agreed to live by certain rules, and although the rules are ignored from time to time we believe the mechanisms of our civilization will restore the balance.

So it is particularly disconcerting when the continual threat of litigation is used as a weapon. It is a perversion of the intent of the law. A legal mechanism of redress, created to protect the rights of all individuals, has been subverted and turned into a lucrative business. The continual threat of malpractice litigation provokes fear in physicians and governs their behavior, irrespective of the actual amount of litigation that occurs in a given state. This is something that every physician knows and recently was demonstrated in a study by Carrier and coworkers reported in *Health Affairs* in 2013. The data showed that the subjective perception of malpractice litigation risk by physicians was reflected directly in their propensity to order diagnostic tests. This ordering of tests did not correlate with the actual amount of litigation. This threat is a substantial psychological burden on physicians, and their response to it—excessive testing and needless referrals—is a much greater actual cost to health care than we appreciate.

On an even more discouraging note, we find that this cancer of fear of malpractice litigation appears to have spread to the medical school curriculum. A report in the *Western Journal of Emergency Medicine* describes third-year medical students' malpractice fear and defensive medicine. Of those in the study, most (82 percent) reported they did not worry about being sued. This is not surprising since they still are in school. However, a majority (56 percent) felt that faculty was concerned about it, and about a third of students believed that faculty taught defensive medicine. About half felt that their enjoyment of medicine would be influenced by malpractice considerations, and about a fourth felt their enjoyment of learning medicine was lessened by malpractice considerations. The venom of the malpractice threat now appears to influence students during a time when they should be engrossed in the beauty and ideals of medicine and learning as much as they can about the proper care of patients.

Medicare relative value units that define the reimbursement for medical and surgical procedures have been described above. However, there may be some benefit to summarizing the concept here in this context. A relative value unit that is used to assign reimbursement for a medical, surgical, or diagnostic procedure has three components: (1) the value of the work done, (2) the expense of carrying out that work, and (3) an allowance for malpractice (usually 2 to 4 percent). There is a fourth component that is often added, and that is the adjustment of payment when the geographic location is considered. A procedure in New York City probably will cost more than one in Des Moines, Iowa, for example.

Contracts are made routinely between service providers and recipients. They define payment for services rendered, and overhead costs and insurance may be included in these. However, I know of no other profession or trade where a value is set for a procedure, and a malpractice allowance is included in the cost of that procedure, independent of the service provider. This is unique to medicine, and its inclusion in the creation of relative value units is an explicit recognition of the vulnerability of physicians to predatory litigation and the widespread prevalence of the practice.

What exactly is defensive medicine? It is a particular variant of defensive decision making, which is the taking of a decision that is not necessarily in the best interests of an organization but is in the best personal interests of those making the decision. This is done frequently in business and politics to avoid a difficult decision that carries consequences if it is incorrect—a decision, by the way, that the persons usually are being well paid to make. It has been estimated that defensive decisions are made in one-third to one-half of instances in some major corporations.

Defensive medical decisions are related to the above but not in the sense that a difficult decision is avoided. That would be morally and ethically indefensible. A physician is expected to evaluate situations that sometimes are confusing yet urgent and then make whatever decision is required. At times these are literally a matter of life and death. The guide is to do what is best for the patient, not what is best for the physician. This is a major distinction from defensive decisions in business and politics. There is no place to hide—as there often is in business or political decisions.

Physicians caring for patients do not have the luxury of dissembling. Combine the need to make explicit decisions about diagnosis or treatment with the background noise of increasing malpractice suits, many of them frivolous, and the encouragement of the patient to litigate if unhappy with the health-care experience or outcome. Would it be a surprise that extra tests were ordered and additional procedures were done; that there might be a tendency to use more technology or newer drugs in order to vitiate a potential later accusation that "not enough was done" to evaluate or treat this patient?

Defensive decision making in medicine generally can be divided into two types: positive (the ordering of additional diagnostic services or additional therapy to deter the patient from filing a malpractice claim by persuading the legal system that the standard of care was met) and negative (practices designed to distance the physician from legal risk by referring the patient elsewhere for further study—a biopsy done by someone else, or referral to a specialist for what will probably be a confirming opinion). Such deviation from good medical practice is induced primarily by a threat of liability and has been invoked as an argument for tort reform for many years. It contributes incrementally to the overuse of health-care services and the overall cost of care.

Defensive medicine has been reported widely in the United States and abroad for many decades. It was described by Hershey in the *Milbank Memorial Fund Quarterly* in 1972, by the US Congress Office of Technology Assessment in 1994, and in a more recent study by Studdert in 2005. Many other examples may be found in the reference sections of the articles just mentioned. It is a reaction to the rising costs of malpractice insurance and increasing likelihood of being sued for a missed or delayed diagnosis or an adverse outcome.

There are very few physicians who will publicly state that they practice defensive medicine—this would leave them open to charges of malpractice from the other direction—but there also are very few physicians who do not practice defensive medicine. The best estimates indicate that about 93 percent of physicians practice defensive medicine. Most of that is by ordering unnecessary diagnostic tests and by referral to other physicians for consultation.

A very good analysis of whether physicians practice defensive medicine and how malpractice reform might change it was presented by Kessler and McClellan in the *Quarterly Journal of Economics* in 1996. It addressed the question of whether fear of liability drives health-care providers to administer treatments or procedures that may not be necessary. They also analyzed the effects of malpractice liability reforms from data taken from Medicare patients treated for serious heart disease over three one-year periods. Their conclusion was clear: malpractice reforms that directly reduce provider liability pressure led to reductions of 5 to 9 percent in medical expenditures *without substantial negative effects on mortality or medical complications.*

An editorial in the *Journal of the American Medical Association* (*JAMA*) by Harris analyzed a study in that same journal that also quantified the costs of defensive medicine from another perspective. During 1983–1984, when malpractice premiums increased enormously, from $1,300 to $8,400 annually, depending upon the specialty, physicians reported changes in their medical practices. This resulted in an average increase of $4,600 in defensive medicine costs per physician per year. From this it could be calculated that each dollar of malpractice risk, measured by insurance premiums, induced $3.50 in defensive medicine expenditures. Thus, the physician who paid $8,400 in premiums was responsible for an additional annual health-care expenditure of $30,000 for defensive medicine.

The thorough and careful study by Studdert and coworkers in 2005 examined defensive medicine practices among high-risk specialist physicians. These included emergency medicine, general surgery, neurosurgery, obstetrics-gynecology, orthopedic surgery, and radiology. All of these are especially affected by fluctuating liability costs. As mentioned, 93 percent reported practicing defensive medicine in one form or another. Many also reported that they had restricted the scopes of their practices because of liability concerns (42 percent) or planned to do so (49 percent).

With respect to the positive type of defensive medicine, 59 percent reported they ordered more diagnostic tests than were medically necessary. The proportion was substantially higher for emergency physicians (70 percent). The most common unnecessary diagnostic test was some form of imaging study.

Negative defensive medicine was reported by 39 percent as well. They stopped caring for high-risk patients. Orthopedic surgeons were more likely to do so (57 percent). Not only were high-risk patients sent elsewhere, patients known to be litigious or to have a greater likelihood of litigating because of the complexity of their clinical problem also were sent elsewhere. Fifty-two percent referred patients to specialists unnecessarily, and this was particularly common among obstetrician-gynecologists (59 percent).

The subjective predictors for all types of defensive medicine were the physicians' confidence in the adequacy of their liability coverage and their perceptions of premium burdens. This study was done in Pennsylvania during a time when insurance companies were dropping malpractice coverage due to the enormous number of lawsuits that were being filed. The situation then in Pennsylvania was far from being unique. Those of us who have lived in Colorado long enough recall in the 1980s that women in Wyoming had to go to Colorado for obstetric care since obstetrician-gynecologists in Wyoming had stopped doing obstetrics due to the enormous cost of malpractice insurance. This occurred not long after many anesthesiologists were driven out of practice by high malpractice premiums, and, as a result, elective surgeries were being delayed across the country. Somehow, this was not enough to bring about tort reform.

Defensive medicine is practiced widely and is a measurable burden as a component of health-care delivery costs. It has the additional effects of imposing enormous psychological strain on the physician, damaging the physician–patient relationship, demeaning the profession of medicine, and confounding the dedication of its practitioners. The quality of medicine suffers, and the conscientious and caring physician begins to think of other things to do in life. As is so often the case, those who want to make a change do not have the power; those with the power will not make the change. Defensive medicine is one of the most damaging yet least recognized alterations in the practice of medicine in the past fifty years.

HUBRIS IN MEDICINE

PHYSICIANS ARE IN A VERY DIFFERENT PLACE NOW AND APPEAR to be innocent bystanders in a disaster that has happened to a vocation that had delivering humans from the bondage of disease as its only raison d'être. That was true whether one practiced clinical medicine or did research. Or, as another physician once said to me, medicine is the only profession that is trying to work itself out of business. People of my vintage went into medicine for what seemed to be all the right reasons. We expected to work long hours, to be at the call of someone in distress, to sacrifice youth to gain knowledge and experience, and to sacrifice time with family to alleviate the suffering of others. I, and my colleagues, if asked, went back to the hospital at night to check on someone or to offer advice; this was considered normal. Given our preoccupation with the welfare of patients, how could we have allowed patients to become products produced by a health-care industry? How were we swept away in the current of profits and quarterly earnings? How did we become irrelevant to the management of health care? Answer: through the natural progression of events in which we were, sequentially, dedicated idealists, haughty intellectuals, detached observers of a declining system, perplexed practitioners, opportunists, gamers of the system, and victims of the system. We may not have been as innocent as we would wish.

I believe it started when physicians, by and large, declined the opportunity to take an active role in the management of hospitals and health care. This was in the early 1960s when medical staffs hired people to manage the hospital. This was done partly in order to devote full time to patient care and partly because it was seen as an unworthy task. "We can hire people to run the hospital. They can't hire people to do what we do," I was told in the course of a conversation about this. "The administrators work for us anyway." Well, that was true and remained so for about a decade thereafter. There were physicians who recognized the importance of bringing medical knowledge and experience in patient care into the management of medical institutions, but they were few and not given credit for the vision they preached. Even these medical administrators perpetuated the more academic approach to medical care that had prevailed for many years. That was perfectly consistent with the times and their backgrounds. The mainstream of physicians, however, remained above it all and continued to practice medicine.

My own introduction into what was to come occurred in the early 1970s, when I was a young faculty member and the new insurance administrator for the Department of Medicine spoke at a faculty luncheon. He was a person who had spent most of his life in the insurance industry and was to lead the department through the billing thickets. It was a lackluster presentation delivered to an uninterested audience. It ended with some advice: if there is a dispute between the physician and the insurance company, "just TWIP it." TWIP was business-speak for "take what insurance pays." Take whatever the payer will give you was not very helpful or prescient, but it gave everyone a path of least resistance to billing issues. It also set the stage for acquiescence to insurance companies in matters of billing. A much later consequence was that insurance companies would decide what procedures, tests, and practices were worth. That put the physician in the unenviable position of importuning a midlevel insurance adjuster for advance permission to use a given procedure, test, or practice for a patient. The American Medical Association, a watchdog for the economics of medicine, saw this and spent much time jousting with the insurance industry over payments. However, the companies set the payments, and then organized medicine had to respond. Medicine had not thought about this in advance since the focus of physicians had been on patient management and not on how to anticipate economic change within the profession—except for personal reimbursement. We were passive during the seventies and eighties as the groundwork was being laid for the domination by insurance companies of medical reimbursement economics and, unfortunately, control of the practice of medicine through control of reimbursement.

One feature that physicians recognized, however, was the fiscal benefits of minimally invasive diagnostic techniques. These included cardiac catheterization with injections of radiopaque dye to measure cardiac function or perfusion of the vascular system; radioisotope injection and radiographic scans of the thyroid, lung, brain, and other organs; endoscopic methods for surgery that permitted smaller incisions, a lower infection rate, and better outcomes; various endoscopes used at either end of the gastrointestinal tract; dialysis machines to manage chronic renal disease; and the many imaging techniques implemented by departments of radiology. It quickly became clear that all of these were reimbursed at higher rates and also were not subject to much argument from the insurance industry. Physicians, being a pragmatic group, began to cluster into those specialties that used these techniques and became proficient with them. Institutions, in their turn, quickly began to seek out specialists who could perform such procedures, paid them well, and billed the public accordingly. This began in the midseventies and grew rapidly through the eighties as radiologists, cardiologists, gastroenterologists, nephrologists, and specialty surgeons came to dominate the ranks of the higher-paid physicians. The demise of general internal medicine, endocrinology, infectious disease, rheumatology, and other specialties—particularly general pediatrics—that did not have access to well-compensated procedures had begun.

I am speaking here, of course, of the economics of medical disciplines and specialties and not of the people in them. Those who had interests in certain areas tended to pursue them without concern about the levels of compensation. However, people are people, and physicians, not surprisingly, are as well. So, if one was not certain of which career path to follow or was equally interested in several specialties, economics certainly could play a role. In addition, if time demands of a specialty were excessive, a change to one where hours were more controllable would be a logical course to follow. Thus, we have seen over the years a decrease in general internists and an increase in dermatologists and radiologists, for example. There now is a shortage of primary care physicians. There has been a decreasing emphasis on self-sacrifice and individualism (and, therefore, a decline in solo practice); an increase in group practice or organizational medicine where hours are predictable; and a steady increase in specialty practice, often built around a technique or procedure of some sort. There is nothing wrong with this, and there is no intent to imply that. It has been a natural progression as ideals of the fifties gave way to the complicated and confusing changes of the sixties, the demands for more ego-centered lifestyles of the seventies, an increasing acceptance of the secular lifestyle and ideals of the eighties, and the rise of the financer or other well-paid executives who managed other people's efforts during the nineties.

This has been the general progression of our society, and it should not be a surprise that children reared in our society should carry those mores of their formative years into medicine as they entered into it. The consequence was that the ideal of the physician in the public and corporate minds underwent a similar change. As the public perceived the shift toward well-paying specialties, fixed hours, and an impersonal insurance reimbursement system that removed the physician from much of the patient–health-care interaction, it was inevitable that the physician as healer, counselor, role model, and advocate of the ill should become shadowed and obscured in the public mind. The magic of medicine was replaced by services provided under more convenient and efficient circumstances and payment extracted by clerks in the office. It was fee for service in the worst sense of that term. This was exactly what was taking place elsewhere in our society, but people elsewhere had not been put on a pedestal because of their knowledge and dedication to the welfare of others. They had no place from which to fall. We followed the movements of society as a whole, since we grew up as its members and, unwittingly, brought those increasingly more secular concepts into medicine.

We all did this, some much more than others. Many simply wanted to practice the art, but the art was increasingly bound to the tyranny of money. When that happens, the art generally is submerged. One can see the beginnings of that today in another area. The university is the last bastion of the intellectual, the independent thinker, the keeper of knowledge. It has steadily increased its costs enormously; prostituted the idea of tenure by giving persons license rather than the liberty to speak the truth—the original concept of tenure; decreased educational standards; and abused its own stature. What alterations are we watching currently in our educational system? The appearance of for-profit universities; increasing use of community colleges; the equating of a college education to job training; cost/benefit comparisons of job training and college; demands to eliminate tenure since it is little more than lifetime job security, which no one else has; an increasing awareness that higher costs have bought a poorer education; and the denigration of the teaching profession in general. Does this not seem like a replay of the ruin of medicine? When the educational system falls, it will be the last of the noble bits of patrimony from a civilization that had its start in the Middle Ages.

Some of the more egregious abusers of the academic medical system were—and remain, I suspect—those faculty members who had positions with tenure and enough influence, based upon their accomplishments and connections, to develop second careers. It was possible to earn a significant amount of money and to live well giving lectures. The "flying professor" who spent much of his time in airplanes while on the lecture tour was a well-recognized entity. Some of this was not only reasonable but also important. One of the charges to academics is not only to create knowledge but also to profess it. This latter is done through publications, lectures in person, and participation at meetings. However, the temptation to expand this into a second, and lucrative, career proved too much for many academicians. The corollary to this was the commercially affiliated academician who not only gave lectures but also had seats on scientific advisory boards or boards of directors and spent much time filling these seats. I met many after I left academic medicine and entered into the executive management of pharmaceutical and biotechnology companies. Few had any commercial experience, but none was short of advice.

A phenomenon of the eighties and, more prominently, the nineties and two thousands was the faculty member who invented or discovered something in the laboratory and formed a company. The technology transfer office of the university, by contract with the faculty member, takes ownership of and patents this discovery and seeks outside capital. The faculty member's focus now may not be medicine, teaching, or patient care; it may become the growth and development of a company in which he or she holds a large number of stock options. The best of both worlds: a salary and benefits guarantee from the university, and stock options from the company. It is a business venture without risk for the founder. The best of the scientists I have known who had such an opportunity passed off the commercial part of the venture to businesspeople and continued to work in their laboratories and clinics. That is in the best spirit of the pursuit of knowledge and the passing on of that knowledge for the betterment of lives.

However, a common path was for the scientific founder of a new company to become an active participant in the commercial development of the company and become immersed in the business. Scientific founders who took control damaged many companies until they were removed or simply ran their businesses into the ground. This probably is the rule rather than the exception. Knowledge of science or medicine is no guarantee of business acumen. But the point here is not academic arrogance but rather the inequity of the situation. The transmutation of an academic career into commercial gain, while retaining all the security of the academic position, has been, in my opinion, one of the worst perversions of academic freedom. I certainly have no quarrel with those who leave academics and enter into the commercial world. That is a change of direction in life and a path available to anyone. But having one's cake and eating it too held medicine and the university up to scorn and provided venture capitalists ingress to the academic system and the corrupting power of money into medicine in general.

All of this, I believe, had a detrimental effect on the appearance of medicine and physicians to the public. The behaviors of some physicians—not the majority or even close to that—who played the system for personal glory or gain cast aspersions on physicians generally. Is there anyone who has not read in the media of certain physicians who are being investigated for Medicare fraud or overbilling of some type or overuse of a particular medical device made by a company in which they have a financial interest? If you think about the numbers, it will become clear that these people are a very small minority of physicians. But the public at large remembers those rather than the physicians who practice good medicine and do not do these things.

A recent event suggests that physicians have been engaged in the fiscal manipulation of medicine long enough now to have embraced the beast. As of this writing, the issue of paying physicians to talk about end-of-life care is being explored. Insurers have begun to reimburse physicians for "advance care planning" conversations. Some stages now cover this for Medicaid patients. The AMA has created billing codes for end-of-life discussions and submitted them to Medicare.

End-of-life planning is very important. It relieves the family and the physician of responsibility for decisions and, as a not unimportant benefit, protects physicians and hospitals from litigation by disgruntled family members. On a more cynical note, insurers are willing and will be increasingly willing to reimburse for time spent on this issue since directions almost always shorten care from full-fledged life-sustaining therapy to something more defined, restrictive, and shorter. This is rationing of health care at the end of life. It was described some years ago as "death-panels" but now is acceptable as the numbers of aging Americans increases and the fiscal implications become clear.

The tragedy in this is the realization that physicians have created reimbursement codes for this. The fiscal reasoning for this is clear, as is the need for explicit end-of-life directives. However, this used to be a responsibility that the physician assumed without billing for it. It was part of the physician–patient relationship, part of the guidance given to patients and families to help at a time of particular crisis. It was not metered and itemized on a bill. It was freely given and was a very human and personal interaction. It was one of the reasons physicians were held in great respect. Have we joined the philistines? Have we become so obsessed with reimbursement issues? It is one thing for insurers to initiate payment for this—it benefits them, and one expects this sort of behavior. It is quite another statement for physicians to create reimbursement codes for this themselves. Unfortunately, this is a consequence of the restrictive time limits for the physician–patient visit. With more time, important human considerations such as this could be woven into the visit. Since medical care now is focused and monitored by the clock, these discussions do not occur. We find ourselves creating reimbursement codes in order to generate a patient visit and receive payment. A few years ago we would have done this as a matter of course. We have fallen further than we know.

All of us were complicit, passively at least, as we acquiesced in our slow disenfranchisement and allowed persons who cared more for business than patient care to manage our institutions and allowed payers whose only concern was the maximization of profit to usurp the revenue side of medical care. We were silent while academic centers became not only sources of knowledge but also headquarters for entrepreneurs who operated risk-free. We now add one final charge, a departure tax, as it were, as our patients leave this world. The effects of all this on medicine are captured by John Donne: "Send not to know for whom the bell tolls, it tolls for thee."

THE REMAINS
OF THE DAY

LIFE CAN ONLY BE UNDERSTOOD
BACKWARDS, BUT IT MUST
BE LIVED FORWARDS.

—Soren Kierkegaard

IF ONE LOOKS AT OUR COST TO DELIVER HEALTH CARE RELATIVE TO
the rest of the world's countries, we have an obvious problem. If
one compares this cost with life expectancy, the picture is even
worse. The comparison in the chart uses international dollars
rather than US dollars. The international dollar is a currency
unit used by international organizations and economists to
compare the values of different currencies around the world.
These are adjusted to reflect currency exchange rates and to
reflect purchasing power parity. This unit represents currencies in
constant dollars for a given base year—or may be extended over
time through adjustment for inflation. This chart is taken from
Global Inequalities in Health Care, a public web page from the
University of California at Santa Cruz.

Using the international dollar metric to simplify comparison,
the graph shows that the United States spends about $4,500 per
capita for a life expectancy of about seventy-seven years. (The
actual US dollar figure is about twice that.) Cuba spends about
11 percent of that for the same life expectancy, and Denmark
has a slightly better life expectancy for 44 percent of our costs.

Consider Canada, with its often-maligned health-care system and a life expectancy substantially more than ours. For that matter, consider almost any European country. Study the graph. It takes only a few moments. Then ask yourself a few questions. Which country spends the most on health care? Which country in the world has the worst cost-benefit ratio for money spent on health care? Which country has a system that rewards big business and insurance companies for managing patients through their various systems at the lowest possible cost to the shareholders? Which country uses quarterly earnings as a metric for efficiency and quality?

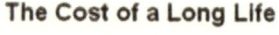

The Cost of a Long Life

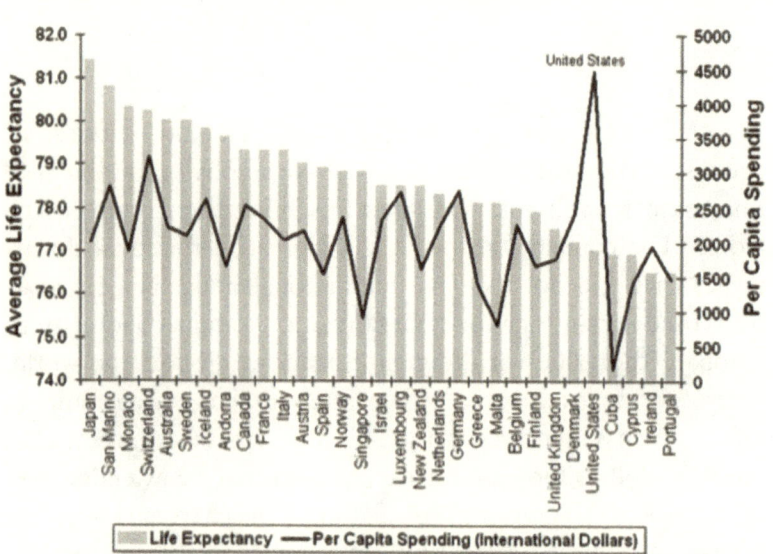

There are many living and economic conditions, styles of living, and forms of government buried in the chart, and one may argue that living in Cuba is far different from living in the United States. That would be true. However, living in Denmark is quite similar to living in the United States, and those in Denmark live quite well at about half our cost.

When one looks at money spent on health care against longevity, there is an enormous disconnect between money spent and years delivered. The United States leaps almost off the chart when compared with the rest of the world, yet we remain at the low end of life expectancy. Lest I be accused of pushing socialism onto the audience, go to the far left of the chart and look at Japan. It has the highest life expectancy and a good style of living, yet its costs to accomplish this are less than half the per capita spending in the United States. The same is true for Switzerland, Israel, Belgium, the United Kingdom, and Germany, to choose other capitalistic and technologically advanced countries, and their costs also are about half of ours for an equal or better life expectancy. This is not due to our use of technology that is driving up the cost; these other countries have access to the same expensive technologies. What these countries have is a single payer system of some type or regulated insurance costs. The argument will be given that these systems are slower, care is not as good, their systems are overburdened, and some elective procedures are delayed inordinately. Much of this is not the case. The major point concerns cost versus benefit. This is driven largely by the profit motive in this country, and it applies to both health-care organizations and insurance companies.

The shift, in our lifetimes, from individual and small group practice to institutional medicine was not necessarily bad. There are many instances of improved efficiency and better patient care. Size is not necessarily a negative factor. The Kaiser Permanente organization, to mention only one of many not-for-profit health-care delivery groups, has done well in caring for patients at a reasonable cost. Coupling medical care with the profit motives of health-care companies and insurance organizations, however, has altered the focus of medical practice from patient care to patient care at the lowest possible cost to the caregiver and payer organizations. The intrusion of these companies into the practice of medicine in order to bring costs to an optimum level certainly is appropriate; demanding some discipline from physicians to be as efficient as possible and to conserve resources also is a reasonable goal. Interfering with good medical care simply to cut costs and increase profits is not.

Until the profit motive is purged from medicine, all talk and action to improve our health-care system will be of little or no benefit. One need only look at health-care systems around the world, each with its own inefficiencies and abuses, to note that the general opinion of consumers is that their country's system is good and benefits all. All of these health-care systems are essentially nonprofit models operated by governments with physicians as employees. Some are single-payer systems, and others are not. These latter use insurance companies, but they are essentially nonprofit as far as health insurance is concerned.

Reid has examined these various health-care systems in his very readable book *The Healing of America*. He explores—by seeking treatment in them—health-care systems in European countries (e.g., France, Germany), the United Kingdom, Canada, Japan, and India. Each of these has a particular type of health-care model that is a variation on a single-payer system or private payer with governmental controls on costs. The exception is India, which has an out-of-pocket payment system that limits health care to those who can afford it. It mimics the system in the United States for those who are not insured. Quality of care is determined by the ability to pay.

The German model uses private care paid for by private insurance; however, there are governmental cost controls that keep costs low. The model in Britain is essentially socialized medicine where the government is the employer and pays all costs. This system is under pressure from costs. The Canadian model is very similar, although the providers are private, and it appears to be reasonably popular. However, there are long waits for some procedures.

According to the author, the United States has systems that follow several of these systems, depending upon population groups. For those not eligible for Medicare, the system is like that in Germany (and Japan), although in the United States the insurance companies are for-profit—a very important difference. For those over sixty-five, our model is similar to that of Canada, in that the government is the payer and care is largely given by the private sector. For the uninsured, care is analogous to that in India: determined by ability to pay.

Each of these has its issues, of course, but they are similar to our own: cost and waiting time for complex treatments. One may seize upon these to show that our system is just as good or better, by pointing out defects. But the fact remains that our costs per capita are exorbitant compared to anywhere in the world, and the profits made by for-profit health-care companies and insurance providers are as well.

Perhaps our benefits are worth the large cost. The relationship between longevity and cost per capita says that this is not the case. Polls taken by the Robert Wood Johnson Foundation, National Public Radio, and the Harvard School of Public Health have found that 87 percent of the general public believes the cost of care is a serious problem. A study from the Institute of Medicine found that about $690 billion are wasted each year in the US health-care system. We are not receiving value for the dollars spent.

Why can we not change the system? Because it comprises 18 percent of the GDP and no one will tamper with it for fear of uncomfortable or egregious economic fallout. It could have been done during the formation of the Affordable Care Act, but it was not. In fact, the behavior of Congress during this charade demonstrates the difficulty of creating the changes that will make a better system for consumers. No politician will touch this. Perhaps the American people are more foresighted than their leaders think.

Could the private sector bring about the needed changes? Let's look at *Strengthening Affordability and Quality in America's Health Care System*, a report published by the Robert Wood Johnson Foundation. It contains five consensus recommendations from the Partnership for Sustainable Health Care. This is a group comprised of consultants from the insurance, hospital, physician, business, and consumer sectors. This group labored and brought forth five recommendations to "control costs and improve the quality of our health care system." The first of these was: "Transform the current payment paradigm by transitioning away from the current fee-for-service payment system towards payment approaches that demonstrate their effectiveness in improving both quality and cost." Can you imagine anything more tepid? Who could argue with that recommendation? Well, no one. Were there solid recommendations as to how to go about doing this? Well, no. Were there any suggestions about reducing the profit motive and using the extra funds to cut the cost of care? Well, again, no.

The second recommendation had something worth considering. "Pay for care that is proven to work by reducing payments for services that prove to be less effective and to have weaker value than alternative therapies." There is something here that could reduce costs by shifting payments based upon quality of care and results. Were there recommendations as to how to do this? There were discussions but no recommendations.

The other three recommendations were bland thoughts, and no one would argue with them either, but they had no substance and no action plans.

This illustrates the problem from the private sector point of view. Consultants brought together to address the problem and suggest ways to improve it will not touch something that is 18 percent of the GDP, just as Congress will not touch it.

In his recent book *Where Does It Hurt?*, Jonathan Bush points out that the number of people supporting each physician has increased from ten in 1990 to sixteen today. Half of these are administrators managing paperwork. This is a 60 percent increase in employment just in one small sector of the health-care delivery system.

For-profit health-care delivery is an enormous business with many competitors. Many industries support these health-care organizations with day-to-day services and supplies. Other industries create, provide, and manage the increasingly complex technology used in health care. The pharmaceutical companies and pharmacy companies create and distribute therapeutic agents. Entire educational systems, from medical schools to community colleges that train lower-level technical and nursing staff, are engaged in supporting the system. The insurance industry that manages payments (and also has the leverage to preapprove or deny medical and surgical therapeutic procedures or treatments) is its own leviathan and an enormous employer that is itself responsible for driving up the cost of care. Finally, all of the individuals who are employed in all of the above are dependent upon the continued functioning of this out-of-control creation for their livelihoods.

There are far too many stakeholders in a system that is not working to consider shutting it down or even to make large changes. Any change will be painful and disruptive, no matter how small. The cost of US health care in 2012 has been calculated at $3 trillion; in 2013, $3.6 trillion; in 2014, $3.8 trillion; and estimated for 2015 at $4 trillion (Forbes, *Pharma and Healthcare*, February 2, 2014, by Dan Munro). There is no real way to constrain it. We have tried to do that every year since about 1985, when the cost was about 11 percent of GDP. There simply are too many people making a living in one way or another from the health-care system. It will continue toward whatever the end will be. As economist Herbert Stein pointed out, "if something cannot go on forever, it will stop." There will be an end, and probably not a pleasant one.

Let us look at this system from another perspective: universal health insurance coverage or the ACA. Set aside for the moment the ineptness of its creation, its fault-ridden introduction, and the new burden on our economy. The ACA did nothing to reduce costs; it shifted them around and undoubtedly will add to them. How we as a nation will fund it remains an important question. These are not small issues, but they are temporary and, with some significant difficulty, will be overcome in the next five to seven years as public demand makes itself felt. The Supreme Court decision to uphold the ACA, the failure of the government shutdown in October 2013 to alter or rescind the ACA, and the general acceptance of the ACA by much of the public all ensure that it is here to stay in one form or another. In fact, the acceptance—embrace even—of the concept of universal coverage by the general public is an indicator that something like this has been needed for a long time in this country. It will provide health care to those who are now uninsured; the care will be more affordable to people individually; there will be more preventive medicine; and there probably will be more emphasis on behavioral change to bring about healthier living. While it will not be the type of care that many of us recall, ultimately it will be a system that provides care to many people who now cannot afford it. Presumably people will no longer become bankrupt because of health-care bills. It is difficult to argue, in concept, against something that will do this.

The general population probably will be better off with the ACA than without it. Spend some time talking with younger people who know little or nothing about medicine of thirty or forty years ago and really do not care about it. They are quite willing to accept governmental involvement if it allows them to save for their children's education. They understand that visits for care are brief and the physician is harried, but it is the system they know. The other thing they know is that they can afford it even though it is more expensive than advertised. In another fifteen years, most of the working population will not know any other form of health-care system. Seven million people have joined, at this writing, and that is a growing endorsement of universal health care.

A study done after the ACA had been in existence for one year demonstrated that it had been successful in achieving some major goals. This study, supported by the Commonwealth Fund, was reported in *Business Insider*. The study showed three things: that the uninsured rate in the US population was dropping, most people like their new insurance, and people are finding it easy to visit a physician. The uninsured rate fell from 20 percent at inception of the ACA to 15 percent after one year. This is a gain of about 9.5 million people either through the exchanges or the expansion of the Medicaid program. The decrease was greatest among the young (10 percent) and Latinos (13 percent); the decrease was disproportionately low among African Americans (1 percent). The law has begun to decrease the uninsured rate among the poor, as was intended. There was a difference among the states that expanded Medicaid (about 11 percent) and those that have not (about 3 percent). Among those newly insured, 58 percent said they were "better off"; among those previously uninsured, 79 percent were "satisfied" or "somewhat satisfied" with the new coverage. Most who gained coverage under the ACA said they could not have accessed care without the new insurance. Finally, about one-fifth of those who signed up have attempted to find a new primary care physician, 75 percent felt the process was "somewhat easy," and two-thirds of these received an appointment within two weeks.

There are the beginnings of success. The unsurprising finding is that US citizens need and want better access to health care. Our historic fee-for-service system has failed them, and the subsequent big-business, high-volume, lower-quality approach has failed them as well. Although the United States probably will not adopt any of the other systems around the world anytime soon, we at least have made a start, inchoate as it is.

The public is relatively indifferent to how the system works or how the physician feels. It just wants a system that provides affordable care in a timely manner. The system that we have now and continue to develop is a variant on *Star Trek* medicine: the physician plays a central role but almost everything is done by technology, paramedical personnel, automation, electronic records, and the computer that manages it all. The physician is the organizer—perhaps "manager" is a more realistic term—and then the synthesizer of the information and, finally, the one who creates the treatment plan. This perhaps is not fundamentally different from the way it was at the half-century mark.

The entry of large business corporations turned the process from one that was centered on providing patient care to one that turned out a product in the shortest possible time and at the lowest cost. The health maintenance organizations in an unholy coupling with insurance companies brought cost-cutting and greed and shifted the burden of increasing quarterly earnings from the corporation onto the physician and patient. As administrative and management personnel and their various directives multiplied, the fixed costs to operate the organizations rose as well. The solution was not to cut out the middle management but rather to task physicians to see more patients (i.e., deliver more product) in less time (i.e., using the assembly line model) with as many standardized protocols as possible.

Recently, it has been suggested that oncologists could treat patients according to standardized protocols rather than individualizing therapy. The sweetener for this would be to pay oncologists additional salary per month to do so—that is, stated differently, provide a thinly disguised bribe to manage patients using predetermined regimens for treating cancers at a time when it is becoming clear to anyone who has paid attention that pharmacogenomics (individualized therapy based upon the genetics of a person's own cancer cells) is a concept that will direct cancer treatment in the near future. Unfortunately, the pernicious effect of money will cause administrators and, worse, may cause chief medical officers as well, to espouse this under the guise of cost-efficient treatment. Medicine has used standardized protocols in managing oncology patients for decades. Some of these have worked well—some childhood leukemias can be cured, as an example—but this is a tumor-specific response. Many other protocols do not work so well, and oncologists continue to search for improvements. Individualized therapy based upon pharmacogenomics is potentially a true breakthrough in oncological treatment. This attempt to return to protocol treatment is an example of what happens when businesspeople decide to interfere in medical therapy. Just as knowledgeable physicians and researchers are moving in one direction, based upon scientific research and clinical data, businesspeople are pushing physicians to move the opposite way, because it will cost less and will be easier for administrators to manage. One wonders about such people.

A related example of the administration interfering with medicine, in this case for marketing reasons, was described in *Emergency Medicine News* recently. In this case, it was the publication on billboards and websites of waiting times in the emergency department (ED)—that may not be so bad if it is a current number that changes as the patient load in the ED fluctuates and simply states the immediate situation. However, many of these are posted as a guarantee and usually are thirty minutes or less. Physicians then are pressured by the administrative system to meet those wait-time guarantees irrespective of the quantity or severity of the patient workload, which, by the very nature of the function of an ED, cannot be predicted over the short term. Moreover, ED visits are increasing as a result of the ACA, and the trend will be an increased use of the ED for the next few years. Some hospitals mandate "greet times," where the physician, regardless of other duties, drops in on a new patient, says "Hello," and returns to the more acute problem. These are, of course, marketing tools and another example of the pernicious effect of big business on the quality of medical care.

Even worse is the fact that some physicians who move to the administrative side of the hospital may become co-opted and forget just what clinical medicine is about. They compound the problem since they carry the weight of the MD degree but are mouthing the slogans and jargon of the businessman. In the above example, a board member of the American College of Emergency Physicians found no fault with trying to speed care in the ED—no argument there—but went on to say, "We need to do what fast-food businesses do—provide a consistent and highly reliable product quickly and to that add our skillful attention, which leads to high quality. Then we can have and give to our patients the best of both worlds." Apparently patients seen in his ED all come in the same size, shape, and degree of acuteness of need and can be managed in the same mindless way in which one turns out hamburgers. This is the noxious effect of business practices and the detrimental effect of administrative interference in medical care. How could a physician lose his touch with medicine and reality so completely? "Do you want morphine with that? Step to the next window."

Other treatment guidelines are being sold to the public and pushed on physicians and lauded in the press as "evidence-based medicine"—as though there is any other kind. These diagnosis and treatment protocols are useful for those who prefer to follow algorithms. The nice thing about algorithms in the management of patients is that there is little thought involved. Anyone can collect a certain amount of patient information, and when there is enough to fill in the blanks on a form, the algorithm will take over to suggest a plan and a treatment. This renders the physician much less important since a lesser-trained person can do this, and it fits well with the business model we reviewed earlier: paramedical personnel seeing more patients in less time. However, the algorithm never will find the outlier diagnosis that will appear on a statistically regular basis, and the paramedical person will not get the nuances of signs and symptoms that raise a lower probability diagnosis to a leading diagnosis. So some patients will not be diagnosed or will be only after an unnecessarily prolonged process. But if one is willing to accept that as a cost of doing business, as we increasingly are, then a certain amount of morbidity and mortality will become the norm.

True evidence-based medicine really is treatment based upon data gleaned from a careful history, physical exam, and diagnostic testing of a particular patient by his or her physician. If there is no physician to do that, then perhaps a prescribed protocol that proscribes original thinking is fine. If the physician is removed from the planning process, and the concept of well-cared-for healthy patients as a goal is deleted from the planning process, then quarterly earnings increases, insurance reimbursement decreases, and maximum patients seen per unit of time will be chosen as the metric with which to measure success. Medicine never was designed for this, it never was intended to be this, physicians never signed up to do this, and no patient wants this. But physicians now are marginalized and will continue to be. This loss of ability to control how therapeutics is done or how patients are managed has frustrated and driven to despair most physicians I know. It is compounded by the knowledge that it will not change. The system is in the grip of for-profit health-care and insurance companies geared to shareholder earnings and executive salaries. Those with the incentive to change the system have no power; those with the power to change it have no incentive. W. B. Yeats described our situation even though he had something else in mind:

> Turning and turning in the widening gyre
> The falcon cannot hear the falconer;
> Things fall apart; the center cannot hold;
> Mere anarchy is loosed upon the world,
> The blood-dimmed tide is loosed, and everywhere
> The ceremony of innocence is drowned;
> The best lack all conviction, while the worst
> Are full of passionate intensity.

CODA AND PERSPECTIVE

THE PRACTICE OF MEDICINE IS AN ART,
NOT A TRADE; A CALLING, NOT A BUSINESS;
A CALLING IN WHICH YOUR HEART WILL
BE EXERCISED EQUALLY WITH YOUR HEAD.

—*Sir William Osler*

LET US LOOK AT THE RESULTANT OF THESE FIFTY YEARS WITH RESPECT to medicine itself, patient care, and the effects on physicians. We shall do it in a vacuum and set aside considerations of the health-care delivery and reimbursement systems.

Many events of these years affected medicine. Much of this was national social change that was massive enough to carry all of us with it. The country moved from the post–World War II calm and order of the fifties into the unanticipated and calamitous social changes of the sixties and early seventies. These questioned virtually every moral and ethical value we espoused personally and as a people. Then it morphed into an increasingly secular society that emerged over about two decades. There was an increase in the presence of government in all aspects of our lives and an economy that rose and fell several times in significant gyrations. The shrinking of our middle class brought about by a shift of wealth into the upper economic class and consequent expansion of the lower made it increasingly obvious that many US citizens could not afford goods and services that had heretofore been accepted as normal—health care being one of these. The great recession of 2008, which came perilously close to a depression, made abundantly clear the need for meaningful regulation of our financial system and the global interconnectedness of our markets and currencies. It served as a catalyst for introduction of universal health care. It also made clear the ineptitude of our political classes and the systems designed to maintain social order.

The technological and scientific revolution completely altered our lives, the conduct of our businesses, and the practice of medicine. Much of this technology had general application, and some was directed specifically to the advancement of medical diagnosis and treatment. At mid-twentieth century, laboratory medicine did not exist. Clinical laboratory testing was slow and done by hand. The development of the autoanalyzer changed this. This surfeit of diagnostic information provided the clinician with much more data than were available before and improved and sped diagnoses. This also helped to change the physician from the source of diagnostic information from accumulated knowledge and experience into the recipient of the information gathered from third parties. Nowhere was this more evident than in radiographic imaging. The X-ray of midcentury gave way at three-quarters of the century to all the imaging methods described. The clinician, through the intermediary of the radiology technician, could look inside the living body and evaluate function.

These advances have given patients access to an ever-better level of scientific medicine: earlier diagnosis and treatment; fewer and less invasive procedures; telemedicine; the tailoring of therapy to genome structure; use of genomics to manage probabilities of diseases; better prenatal diagnosis and therapy; and new applications of robotic surgery. Regenerative medicine will provide new tissues and, ultimately, new organs. Science and technology have moved medicine forward logarithmically. We do things now as a matter of course that were undreamed of at midcentury. Patients now are very fortunate. How about physicians? We are much better off as well. The benefits of technology have provided us with the tools and knowledge to diagnose more accurately and treat more diseases more efficiently. We are very fortunate to have access to these advances.

It is perhaps not too far-fetched to draw an analogy here. In the Middle Ages, the writings of Copernicus and Galileo challenged the harmony of the spheres and destroyed the earth-centric universe. Later, Newton would describe the mathematics of gravity and the way it managed the orbits of the planets. Still later, the continuing increase in knowledge and science would bring about the age of reason. All this, with its attendant social change, took place over a relatively few centuries. As art, mystery, and authority gave way to science, mechanism, and challenge, there was a decline in the influence of religion and the priestly caste along with a concomitant elevation of a new caste: the scientist and inventor. Not far behind were the industrial entrepreneurs who risked much and profited greatly from the discoveries and new knowledge.

Something very similar occurred in medicine, but it did not take centuries; it took only a few decades of the past half century and was largely due to the influence of computers and the rapid dissemination of information. The relationship of physician and patient was not too far, conceptually, from that of the priest and supplicant. Then, over the course of a few decades, the art of medicine was replaced by the science and technology of medicine with the addition of many technical and ancillary people. The physician was slowly reduced from Magister Ludi—whose inherent diagnostic insight was the magic of the art and whose devotion to and intellectual absorption in medicine was his undoing—to manager of the team who integrated information and dispensed the therapy according to the results of the technological testing sequence.

As science and reason replaced religion and philosophy in the fifteenth to eighteenth centuries, there was uncertainty in the minds of people as to their place in the universe and eternity. Similarly, as the hierarchical physician-to-underling relationship began to disintegrate, there was uncertainty in the minds of physicians as to their roles. People who sought medical attention also became unsure about where to go to obtain healing as the visible role of the physician declined, costs increased, people were priced out of medical care by exorbitant fees for service, and business debased what had been an intensely personal relationship. The pseudoscience that grew to fill the vacuum offered new, and untried, treatment options, cures, and offers of healing to a society that had undergone a revolution in its thinking. This new industry—the word is appropriate here—promised healing that was based more on hope than science. The current businesses of therapeutics using vitamins, nutritional supplements, and nostrums of all sorts, along with the many givers of advice on television and other media, are the visible evidence of this decline in the influence of medicine. Once the faith in a path is broken, untried but seemingly attractive newer paths will be offered. Many rush to try them and, once converted, become zealots. The placebo effect, which is surprisingly strong, underpins this phenomenon. These are not cures, but the person believes them to be, and that is often enough to assure success. As frivolous and wasteful of time and money as many of these are, at least they are largely innocuous. The exception to this is the path of therapeutic nihilism, which discards vaccines. This willful ignorance in a society that has taken the advice to "do your own thing" from the sixties and carried it forward has produced whooping cough epidemics in this country almost a century after the unarguable benefits of vaccines were made clear. This is a tragedy for those children made to suffer for their parents' ignorance. When pseudoscience and science occupy the same space, advertising and gossip generally win the day.

An increasingly complex therapeutic system requires an increasingly complex variety of providers. Physicians now are only one of these. They have become decreasingly the guides and guardians of the health-care system and are now supervisors in the mosaic of provision of care. Although I find a personal health-care visit to be a sterile interaction, I cannot deny that it is more efficient and more effective than the medicine we practiced. Our model has gone, and another has taken its place. The improvements in technology and, more recently, in the payment systems that now protect more people are greatly to the benefit of patients.

The tragedy in the past half century is that the astounding improvements in technology cost us the human touch. Had that been retained, we truly would have the best of all possible worlds. This loss is due almost completely to the intrusion of corporate business practices in the health-care and insurance industries. Perhaps some of the blame also resides with physicians. We could have tried harder to keep the system from disenfranchising both patients and physicians, but I think we did not really see where things were going until too late. It may be that physicians can reclaim something of their former positions by returning to earlier habits: by working for something larger than themselves. They can, as no one else can, serve as patient advocates and educators in a system that deals with patients as ciphers. Physicians also can educate the public to counter direct advertising about drugs and talk show misinformation. This would require a conscious change in attitude and a rededication to the physician–patient relationship as it once was—tempered, to be sure, with the realities of the present. This attitude change would communicate itself rather quickly to the patient, and what was a brief by-the-clock encounter would become a brief by-the-clock personal encounter. This could be done with the extra question about family, some advice beyond drugs or surgical procedures, and the kinds of human inquiries that we all appreciate but which are largely absent from current patient encounters. Physicians still are shocked by what has occurred and cowed by the pronouncements that come from the corporate philistines in charge of health care.

Two-thirds of the population recognizes the high cost of care as a very serious problem for the country. Physicians, individually and collectively must speak out against these costs and advocate measures to mitigate them. A demonstration by the medical profession that it is as appalled by the changes in health care as is the general public would go far toward restoring the public trust in physicians. Fifty years ago we were accustomed to speaking out against injustice and expressing our opinions openly. When did we become so passive and pliable? Are we as concerned about money and perquisites as those in the corporate suites? Let us hope not and begin to behave accordingly.

The system will not change, but injections of humanity into it from the medical community would go far toward improving what we have. I have no doubt that patients would welcome this as well. Most of us believe that the human being is more than biology. This may be for religious reasons or simply because we are unwilling to write ourselves off as equivalent to a dog, fish, or palm tree. We make ethical and moral judgments, we plan, we pursue dreams, we comprehend beauty, and we think in the abstract. We are some blend of the material and the mysterious. Most of us do not think of ourselves as products of a health-care system. The interaction of a human with a problem and a physician who attempts to heal is one of the most human and personal of relationships. It does not lend itself to accounting ledgers, quarterly earnings postings, and visits per hour. It is more than that.

The physician still is here, although we practice differently. We play a very important and essential role, but it will be increasingly a supervisory role. Can you imagine a physician supervising a cadre of physician assistants or nurse practitioners in lieu of individual family physicians? How about a surgeon managing several operations performed by skilled technicians or robots? Not only can I imagine all of these, they are beginning to occur. In our own minds, we have been marginalized; in the minds of patients, we still are here. In fact, they would like us to play a larger role since they are as aware as we of the impersonal nature of the health-care visit. We remain very much in the game and could make the visits more personal if we try. We perhaps can change the sensitivity of the system from within even though we can no longer change its structure.

REFERENCES

THE WAY WE WERE

Duffy, T. P. "The Flexner Report—100 Years Later." *Yale Journal of Biology and Medicine* 84, no. 3 (2011): 269–76.

EXPANSION OF THE MEDICAL CARE SYSTEM

Callans, D. "Out-of-Hospital Cardiac Arrest—The Solution Is Shocking." *New England Journal of Medicine* 351, no. 7 (2004): 632–34.

Edgerly, D. "Birth of EMS: The History of the Paramedic." *Journal of Emergency Medical Services* (October 8, 2013). http://www.jems.com.

Goodman, L., and T. Norbeck. "Who's to Blame for Our Rising Healthcare Costs?" *Forbes*, April 3, 2013. http://www.forbes.com/sites/realspin/2013/04/03/whos-to-blame-for-our-rising-healthcare-costs/.

Pope, A. *The Poetical Works of Alexander Pope.* New York: Thomas Y. Crowell, 1896.

Schroeder, S. A. "Personal Reflections on the High Cost of American Medical Care: Many Causes but Few Politically Sustainable Solutions." *Archives of Internal Medicine* 171, no. 8 (2011): 722–27. doi: 10.1001/archinternmed.2011.149.

Social Security Administration. "History of SSA During the Johnson Administration 1963–1968." Accessed

November 9, 2014. http://www.ssa.gov/history/ssa/lbjmedicare4.html.

The Advent and Dominance of Technology

Best, W. R. "The Potential Role of Computers in Medical Practice." *Journal of the American Medical Association* 182, no. 10 (1962): 994–1000.

Caceres, C. A. "Electrographic Analysis by a Computer System." *Archives of Internal Medicine* 111, no. 2 (1963): 196–201.

Medical News. "An 'On-the-Spot' 4-Second ECG Analysis." *Journal of the American Medical Association* 183, no. 24 (1963).

Williams, G. Z. "Clinical Pathology Tomorrow." *American Journal of Clinical Pathology* 37, February (1962): 121–24.

——— "Effects of Automation on Laboratory Diagnosis." *California Medicine* 108, January, (1968): 43–45.

Administration of Medicine

Mathews, Anna Wilde, and Tom McGinty. "Physician Panel Prescribes the Fees Paid by Medicare." *The Wall Street Journal*, October 26, 2010. http://online.wsj.com/articles/SB100014240527487046573045755404401773772102.

Crisp, N., and L. Chen. "Global Supply of Health Professionals." *New England Journal of Medicine* 370 (2014): 950–57.

Hsiao, W. C., et al. "Results and Policy Implications of the Resource-Based Relative-Value Study." *New England Journal of Medicine* 319, no. 13 (1988): 881–88.

Reinhardt, Uwe. "How Medicare Pays Physicians." *The New York Times*, December 6, 2010. http://exonomix.blogs.nytimes.com 2010/12/03/.

——— "The Little-Known Decision-Makers for Medicare Physicans Fees." *The New York Times*, December 10, 2010. http://exonomix.blogs.nytimes.com /2010/12/10/.

For-Profit and Nonprofit

Davis, K., and J. Ballreich. "Equitable Access to Care—How the United States Ranks Internationally." *New England Journal of Medicine* 371, no. 17 (2014): 1567–70.

Horwitz, J. R. "Making Profits and Providing Care: Comparing Nonprofit, For-Profit, and Government Hospitals." *Health Affairs (Millwood)* 24, no. 3 (2005): 790–801.

Roomkin, M. J., and B. A. Weisbrod. "Managerial Compensation and Incentives in For-Profit and Nonprofit Hospitals." *Journal of Law, Economics, & Organization* 15 (1999): 750–781.

Shaywitz, D. A. Review of *Where Does It Hurt?*, by J. Bush and S. Baker. *Wall Street Journal*, May 19, 2014.

Singh, H., A. N. Meyer, and E. J. Thomas. "The Frequency of Outpatient Diagnostic Errors: Estimations from Three Large Observational Studies Involving US Adult Populations." *BMJ Quality and Safety* 23, no. 9 (2014): 727–31. doi: 10.1136/bmjqs-2013-002627.

Ubel, P. "Is the Profit Motive Ruining American Healthcare?" Pharma and Health Care. *Forbes*, February 12, 2014. http://www.forbes.com/sites/peterubel/2014/02/12/is-the-profit-motive-ruining-american-healthcare/.

Zane, F. P. "The Bureaucrat Sitting on Your Doctor's Shoulder: When I'm operating on a child, I shouldn't have to wonder if Medicaid will OK a change in the surgical plan." *Wall Street Journal*, Thursday, May 22, 2014: A13.

Defensive Medicine

Baker, P. "Bush Campaigns to Curb Lawsuits." *Washington Post*, January 6, 2005: A6.

Carrier, E. R., J. D. Reschovsky, D. A. Katz, and M. M. Mello. "High Physician Concern about Malpractice Risk Predicts More Aggressive Diagnostic Testing In Office-Based Practice." *Health Affairs* 32, no. 8 (2013): 1383–91.

Chief Medical Officer, National Health Service. "Making Amends: A Consultation Paper Setting Out Proposals for Reforming the Approach to Clinical Negligence in the NHS." Leeds, United Kingdom: Department of Health, June 2003.

Dao, J. "A Push in States to Curb Malpractice Costs." *New York Times*, January 14, 2005: A21.

Emanuel, E. J. "What Cannot Be Said on Television about Health Care." *Journal of the American Medical Association* 297, no. 19 (2007): 21–31.

Emanuel, E. J., and V. R. Fuchs. "The Perfect Storm of Overutilization." *Journal of the American Medical Association* 299, no. 23 (2008): 2789–91.

Glassman, P. A., J. E. Rolph, L. P. Petersen, M. A. Bradley, and R. L. Kravitz. "Physicians' Personal Malpractice Experiences Are Not Related to Defensive Clinical Practices." *Journal of Health Politics, Policy and Law* 21, no. 2 (1996): 219–41.

Hagihara A., M. Nishi, and K. Nobutomo. "Standard of Care and Liability in Medical Malpractice Litigation in Japan." *Health Policy* 65 (2003): 119–27.

Harris, J. E. "Defensive Medicine: It Costs, but Does It Work?" *Journal of the American Medical Association* 257, no. 20 (1987): 2801–2.

Hershey, N. "The Defensive Practice of Medicine: Myth or Reality." *Milbank Memorial Fund Quarterly* July, 50, no. 3 (1972): 69–98.

Ipp, D. A., P. Cane, D. Sheldon, and I. Macintosh. *Review of the Law of Negligence: Final Report.* Canberra, Australia: Commonwealth of Australia, September 2002.

Johnston, W. F., R. M. Rodriguez, D. Suarez, and B. S. Fortman. "Study of Medical Students' Malpractice Fear and Defensive Medicine." *Western Journal of Emergency Medicine* 15, no. 3 (2014): 293–98.

Kessler, D., and M. McClelland. "Do Doctors Practice Defensive Medicine?" *Quarterly Journal of Economics* 111, no. 2 (1996): 353–90.

Studdert, D. M., M. M. Mello, W. M. Sage, C. M. DesRoches, J. Peugh, K. Zapert, and T. A. Brennan. "Defensive Medicine among High-Risk Specialist Physicians in a Volatile Malpractice Environment." *Journal of the American Medical Association* 293, no. 21 (2005): 2609–17.

Studdert, D. M., M. M. Mello, A. A. Gawande, T. K. Gandhi, A. Kachalia, C. Yoon, A. L. Puopolo, and T. A. Brennan. "Claims, Errors, and Compensation Payments in Medical Malpractice Litigation." *New England Journal of Medicine.* May 11; 354, no. 19 (2006): 2024–33.

Summerton, N. "Positive and Negative Factors in Defensive Medicine." *BMJ,* January 7; 310, no. 6971 (1995): 27–29.

US Congress; Office of Technology Assessment. *Defensive Medicine and Medical Malpractice.* Washington, DC: US Government Printing Office, 1994. Publication OTA-H-602.

Veldhuis, M. "Defensive Behavior of Dutch Family Physicians: Widening the Concept." *Family Medicine* 26, no. 1 (1994): 27–29.

THE REMAINS OF THE DAY

Blendon, R. J., J. M. Benson, and J. O. Hero. "Public Trust in Physicians—US Medicine in International Perspective." *New England Journal of Medicine* 371, no. 17 (2014): 1570–72.

Bush, J., and S. Baker. *Where Does It Hurt? An Entrepreneur's Guide to Fixing Health Care.* New York: Portfolio, 2014.

Eastaugh, S. R. "Managing Risk in a Risky World." *Journal of Health Care Finance* 25, no. 3 (1999): 17–21.

LoGiurato, B. "Major New Study Says Obamacare Is Working—Even for Republicans." *Business Insider,*

July 10, 2014. http://www.businessinsider.com/ study-obamacare-reduces-uninsured-rate-2014-7.

Reid, T. R. *The Healing of America: A Global Quest for Better, Cheaper, and Fairer Health Care.* New York: Penguin Press, 2010.

Scheck, A. "A Special Report: Wait-Time Estimates: Patient Care Advance or Marketing Strategy?" *Emergency Medicine News* 36, no. 7 (2014): 14–15.

University of California, Santa Cruz. "Global Inequalities in Health." http://ucatlas.ucsc.edu/health.php.

Yeats, W. B. *The Second Coming.* Scribner,New York, 1996.

TRUE DIRECTIONS
An affiliate of Tarcher Books

OUR MISSION

Tarcher's mission has always been to publish books
that contain great ideas. Why? Because:

GREAT LIVES BEGIN WITH GREAT IDEAS

At Tarcher, we recognize that many talented authors, speakers,
educators, and thought-leaders share this mission and deserve to be
published – many more than Tarcher can reasonably publish ourselves.
True Directions is ideal for authors and books that increase awareness,
raise consciousness, and inspire others to live their ideals and passions.

Like Tarcher, True Directions books are designed to do three things:
inspire, inform, and motivate.

Thus, True Directions is an ideal way for these important voices
to bring their messages of hope, healing, and help to the world.

Every book published by True Directions– whether it is non-
fiction, memoir, novel, poetry or children's book – continues
Tarcher's mission to publish works that bring positive change
in the world. We invite you to join our mission.

For more information, see the True Directions website:
www.iUniverse.com/TrueDirections/SignUp

Be a part of Tarcher's community to bring positive change in this world!
See exclusive author videos, discover new and exciting books, learn about
upcoming events, connect with author blogs and websites, and more!
www.tarcherbooks.com

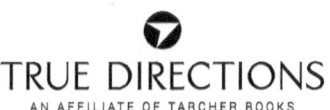

TRUE DIRECTIONS
AN AFFILIATE OF TARCHER BOOKS